Virtual Clinical Excursions—Psychiatric

for

Stuart and Laraia:
Principles and Practice of Psychiatric Nursing,
8th Edition

Virtual Clinical Excursions—Psychiatric

for

Stuart and Laraia:
Principles and Practice of Psychiatric Nursing,
8th Edition

prepared by

Susan Fertig McDonald, MSN, RN, CS
Clinical Nurse Specialist—Psychiatry
VA San Diego Healthcare System
San Diego, California

software developed by

Wolfsong Informatics, LLC
Tucson, Arizona

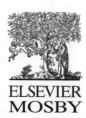

ELSEVIER
MOSBY

ELSEVIER
MOSBY

11830 Westline Industrial Dr.
St. Louis, Missouri 63146

VIRTUAL CLINICAL EXCURSIONS—PSYCHIATRIC FOR
STUART AND LARAIA: PRINCIPLES AND PRACTICE OF
PSYCHIATRIC NURSING,
EIGHTH EDITION

ISBN 0-323-03042-4

Copyright © 2006, Mosby, Inc.

Notice

Knowledge and best practice in this field are constantly changing. As new research and experience broaden our knowledge, changes in practice, treatment and drug therapy may become necessary or appropriate. Readers are advised to check the most current information provided (i) on procedures featured or (ii) by the manufacturer of each product to be administered, to verify the recommended dose or formula, the method and duration of administration, and contraindications. It is the responsibility of the practitioner, relying on their own experience and knowledge of the patient, to make diagnoses, to determine dosages and the best treatment for each individual patient, and to take all appropriate safety precautions. To the fullest extent of the law, neither the Publisher nor the Authors assumes any liability for any injury and/or damage to persons or property arising out or related to any use of the material contained in this book.

International Standard Book Number 0-323-03042-4

Senior Editor, Nursing: *Tom Wilhelm*
Managing Editor: *Jeff Downing*
Associate Developmental Editor: *Jennifer Anderson*
Project Manager: *Joy Moore*

Printed in the United States of America

Last digit is the print number: 9 8 7 6 5 4 3 2 1

*Workbook
prepared by*

Susan Fertig McDonald, MSN, RN, CS
Clinical Nurse Specialist—Psychiatry
VA San Diego Healthcare System
San Diego, California

Textbook

Gail Wiscarz Stuart, PhD, APRN, BC, FAAN
Dean and Professor, College of Nursing
Professor, College of Medicine
Department of Psychiatry and Behavioral Sciences
Medical University of South Carolina
Charleston, South Carolina

Michele T. Laraia, PhD, RN, CS
Associate Professor
Director, Advanced Practice Nursing Programs
School of Nursing
Oregon Health and Science University
Portland, Oregon

Contents

Table of Contents
Stuart and Laraia:
Principles and Practice of Psychiatric Nursing, 8th Edition

Getting Started

GETTING SET UP

■ MINIMUM SYSTEM REQUIREMENTS

WINDOWS™

Windows XP, 2000, 98, ME, NT 4.0 (Recommend Windows XP/2000)
Pentium® III processor (or equivalent) @ 600 MHz (Recommend 800 MHz or better)
128 MB of RAM (Recommend 256 MB or more)
800 x 600 screen size (Recommend 1024 x 768)
Thousands of colors
12x CD-ROM drive
Soundblaster 16 soundcard compatibility
Stereo speakers or headphones

Note: Virtual Clinical Excursions—Psychiatric for Windows will require a minimal amount of disk space to install icons and required dll files for Windows 98/ME.

MACINTOSH®

MAC OS X (10.2 or higher)
Apple Power PC G3 @ 500 MHz or better
128 MB of RAM (Recommend 256 MB or more)
800 x 600 screen size (Recommend 1024 x 768)
Thousands of colors
12x CD-ROM drive
Stereo speakers or headphones

■ INSTALLATION INSTRUCTIONS

WINDOWS

1. Insert the *Virtual Clinical Excursions—Psychiatric* CD-ROM.
2. Inserting the CD should automatically bring up the setup screen if the current product is not already installed.
   a. If the setup screen does not appear automatically (and *Virtual Clinical Excursions—Psychiatric* has not been installed already), navigate to the "My Computer" icon on your desktop or in your Start menu.
   b. Double-click on your CD-ROM drive.
   c. If installation does not start at this point:
      (1) Click the **Start** icon on the task bar and select the **Run** option.
      (2) Type d:\setup.exe (where "d:\" is your CD-ROM drive) and press **OK**.
      (3) Follow the onscreen instructions for installation.
3. Follow the onscreen instructions during the setup process.

MACINTOSH

1. Insert the *Virtual Clinical Excursions—Psychiatric* CD in the CD-ROM drive. The disk icon will appear on your desktop.
2. Double-click on the disk icon.
3. Double-click on the PSYCHIATRIC_MAC run file.

NOTE: *Virtual Clinical Excursions—Psychiatric* for Macintosh does not have an installation setup and can only be run directly from the CD.

■ HOW TO USE VIRTUAL CLINICAL EXCURSIONS—PSYCHIATRIC

WINDOWS

1. Double-click on the *Virtual Clinical Excursions—Psychiatric* icon located on your desktop.
2. Or navigate to the program via the Windows Start menu.

NOTE: Windows 98/ME will require you to restart your computer before running the *Virtual Clinical Excursions—Psychiatric* program.

MACINTOSH

1. Insert the *Virtual Clinical Excursions—Psychiatric* CD in the CD-ROM drive. The disk icon will appear on your desktop.
2. Double-click on the disk icon.
3. Double-click on the PSYCHIATRIC_MAC run file.

■ SCREEN SETTINGS

For best results, your computer monitor resolution should be set at a minimum of 800 x 600. The number of colors displayed should be set to "thousands or higher" (High Color or 16 bit) or "millions of colors" (True Color or 24 bit).

Windows™

1. From the **Start** menu, select **Control Panel** (on some systems, you will first go to **Settings**, then to **Control Panel**).
2. Double-click on the **Display** icon.
3. Click on the **Settings** tab.
4. Under **Screen area** use the slider bar to select **800 by 600 pixels**.
5. Access the **Colors** drop-down menu by clicking on the down arrow.
6. Select **High Color (16 bit)** or **True Color (24 bit)**.
7. Click on **OK**.
8. You may be asked to verify the setting changes. Click **Yes**.
9. You may be asked to restart your computer to accept the changes. Click **Yes**.

Macintosh®

1. Select the **Monitors** control panel.
2. Select **800 x 600** (or similar) from the **Resolution** area.
3. Select **Thousands** or **Millions** from the **Color Depth** area.

■ WEB BROWSERS

Supported web browsers include Microsoft Internet Explorer (IE) version 5.0 or higher and Netscape version 4.5 or higher. *Note that Netscape version 6.0 is not supported at this time, although versions 6.2 and higher are supported.*

If you use America Online (AOL) for web access, you will need AOL version 4.0 or higher and IE 5.0 or higher. Do not use earlier versions of AOL with earlier versions of IE, because you will have difficulty accessing many features.

For best results with AOL:
- Connect to the Internet using AOL version 4.0 or higher.
- Open a private chat within AOL (this allows the AOL client to remain open, without asking whether you wish to disconnect while minimized).
- Minimize AOL.
- Launch a recommended browser.

■ TECHNICAL SUPPORT

Technical support for this product is available between 7:30 a.m. and 7 p.m. CST, Monday through Friday. Before calling, be sure that your computer meets the minimum system requirements to run this software. Inside the United States and Canada, call 1-800-692-9010. Outside North America, call 314-872-8370. You may also fax your questions to 314-997-5080 or contact Technical Support through e-mail: technical.support@elsevier.com.

Trademarks: Windows, Macintosh, Pentium, and America Online are registered trademarks.

ACCESSING *Virtual Clinical Excursions—Psychiatric* FROM EVOLVE ───────────────

The product you have purchased is part of the Evolve family of online courses and learning resources. Please read the following information completely to get started.

To access your instructor's course on Evolve:

Your instructor will provide you with the username and password needed to access their specific course on the Evolve Learning System. Once you have received this information, please follow these instructions:

1. Go to the Evolve student page (http://evolve.elsevier.com/student)

2. Enter your username and password in the **Login to My Evolve** area and click the **Login** button.

3. You will be taken to your personalized **My Evolve** page where the course will be listed in the **My Courses** module.

TECHNICAL REQUIREMENTS

To use an Evolve course, you will need access to a computer that is connected to the Internet and equipped with web browser software that supports frames. For optimal performance, it is recommended that you have speakers and use a high-speed Internet connection. However, slower dial-up modems (56 K minimum) are acceptable.

Whichever browser you use, the browser preferences must be set to enable cookies and Java/JavaScript and the cache must be set to reload every time.

Enable Cookies

Browser	Steps
Internet Explorer 5.0 or higher	1. Select **Tools**. 2. Select **Internet Options**. 3. Select **Security** tab. 4. Make sure **Internet** (globe) is highlighted. 5. Select **Custom Level** button. 6. Scroll down the **Security Settings** list. 7. Under **Cookies** heading, make sure **Enable** is selected. 8. Click **OK**.
Internet Explorer 6.0	1. Select **Tools**. 2. Select **Internet Options**. 3. Select **Privacy** tab. 4. Use the slider (slide down) to **Accept All Cookies**. 5. Click **OK**. -OR- 4. Click the **Advanced** button. 5. Click the check box next to **Override Automatic Cookie Handling**. 6. Click the **Accept** buttons under **First-party Cookies** and **Third-party Cookies**. 7. Click **OK**.
Netscape Communicator or Navigator 4.5 or higher	1. Select **Edit**. 2. Select **Preferences**. 3. Click **Advanced**. 4. Click **Accept all cookies**. 5. Click **OK**.
Netscape Communicator or Navigator 6.1 or higher	1. Select **Edit**. 2. Select **Preferences**. 3. Select **Privacy & Security**. 4. Select **Cookies**. 5. Select **Enable All Cookies**.

Enable Java

Browser	Steps
Internet Explorer 5.0 or higher	1. Select **Tools**. 2. Select **Internet Options**. 3. Select the **Advanced** tab. 4. Locate **Microsoft VM**. 5. Make sure the **Java console enabled** and **Java logging enabled** boxes are checked. 6. Click **OK**. 7. Restart your computer if you checked the **Java console enabled** box.
Netscape Communicator or Navigator 4.5 or higher	1. Select **Edit** 2. Select **Preferences**. 3. Select **Advanced**. 4. Make sure the **Enable Java** and **Enable JavaScript** boxes are checked. 5. Click **OK**.

Set Cache to Always Reload a Page

Browser	Steps
Internet Explorer 5.0 or higher	1. Select **Tools**. 2. Select **Internet Options**. 3. Select the **General** tab. 4. Select **Settings** from within the **Temporary Internet Files** section. 5. Select the **Every visit to the page** button. 6. Click **OK**.
Netscape Communicator or Navigator 4.5 or higher	1. Select **Edit** 2. Select **Preferences**. 2. Click the **+** or **→** icon next to the **Advanced** to see more options. 3. Select **Cache**. 4. Select the **Every time** button at the bottom. 5. Click **OK**.

Plug-Ins

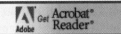

Adobe Acrobat Reader—With the free Acrobat Reader software you can view and print Adobe PDF files. Many Evolve products offer student and instructor manuals, checklists, and more in this format!

Download at: http://www.adobe.com

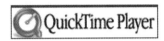

Apple QuickTime—Install this to hear word pronunciations, heart and lung sounds, and many other helpful audio clips within Evolve Online Courses!

Download at: http://www.apple.com

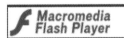

Macromedia Flash Player—This player will enhance your viewing of many Evolve web pages, as well as educational short-form to long-form animation within the Evolve Learning System!

Download at: http://www.macromedia.com

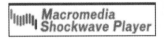

Macromedia Shockwave Player—Shockwave is best for viewing the many interactive learning activities within Evolve Online Courses!

Download at: http: //www.macromedia.com

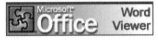

Microsoft Word Viewer—With this viewer Microsoft Word users can share documents with those who don't have Word, and users without Word can open and view Word documents. Many Evolve products have testbank, student and instructor manuals, and other documents available for downloading and viewing on your own computer!

Download at: http://www.microsoft.com

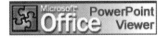

Microsoft PowerPoint Viewer—View PowerPoint 97, 2000, and 2002 presentations even if you don't have PowerPoint with this viewer. Many Evolve products have slides available for downloading and viewing on your own computer!

Download at: http://www.microsoft.com

SUPPORT INFORMATION

Live support is available to customers in the United States and Canada from 7:30 a.m. to 7:00 p.m. (Central Time), Monday through Friday by calling, **1-800-401-9962**. You can also send an email to evolve-support@elsevier.com.

There is also **24/7 support information** available on the Evolve website (http://evolve.elsevier.com), including:

- Guided Tours
- Tutorials
- Frequently Asked Questions (FAQs)
- Online Copies of Course User Guides
- And much more!

A QUICK TOUR

Welcome to *Virtual Clinical Excursions—Psychiatric*, a virtual hospital setting in which you can work with multiple complex patient simulations and also learn to access and evaluate the information resources that are essential for high-quality patient care.

The virtual hospital, Pacific View Regional Hospital, has realistic architecture and access to patient rooms, a Nurses' Station, and a Medication Room.

■ BEFORE YOU START

Make sure you have your textbook nearby when you use the *Virtual Clinical Excursions—Psychiatric* CD. You will want to consult topic areas in your textbook frequently while working with the CD and using this workbook.

■ HOW TO SIGN IN

- Enter your name on the Student Nurse identification badge.
- Next, click the down arrow next to **Select Floor**. This drop-down menu lists only the floors on which there are currently patients with psychiatric nursing needs: Medical-Surgical, Obstetrics, Pediatrics, and Skilled Nursing. (For this quick tour, choose **Obstetrics**.)
- Now click the down arrow next to **Select Period of Care**. This drop-down menu gives you four periods of care from which to choose. In Periods of Care 1 through 3, you can actively engage in patient assessment, entry of data in the electronic patient record (EPR), and medication administration. Period of Care 4 presents the day in review; during this shift, you can access all records, but you cannot visit patients in their rooms. Highlight and click the appropriate period of care. (For this quick tour, choose **Period of Care 2**.)
- Click **Go** in the lower right side of the screen.
- This takes you to the Patient List screen (see example on page 11). Only the patients on the floor you choose (e.g., Obstetrics) are available. Note that the virtual time is provided in the box at the lower left corner of the screen (0730, since we chose Period of Care 1).

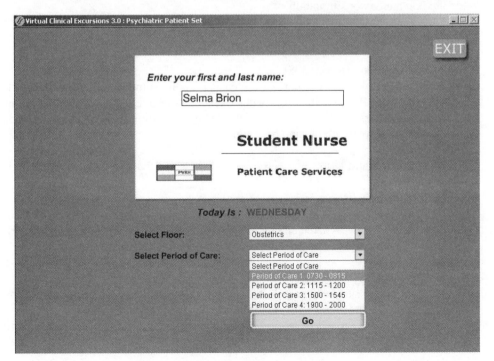

■ PATIENT LIST

MEDICAL-SURGICAL UNIT

Harry George (Room 401)
Osteomyelitis—A middle-age Caucasian male admitted from a homeless shelter with an infected leg. He has complications of type 2 diabetes mellitus, alcohol abuse, nicotine addiction, poor pain control, and complex psychosocial issues.

Jacquline Catanazaro (Room 402)
Asthma—A middle-age Caucasian female admitted with an acute asthma exacerbation and suspected pneumonia. She has complications of chronic schizophrenia, noncompliance with medication therapy, obesity, and herniated disc.

OBSTETRICS UNIT

Dorothy Grant (Room 201)
30-week intrauterine pregnancy—A young Caucasian multipara admitted with abdominal trauma following a domestic violence incident. Her complications include preterm labor and extensive social issues such as acquiring safe housing for her family upon discharge.

Kelly Brady (Room 203)
26-week intrauterine pregnancy—A middle-age Caucasian primigravida urgently admitted for progressive symptoms of preeclampsia. A history of inadequate coping with major life stressors leave her at risk for a recurrence of depression as she faces a diagnosis of HELLP syndrome and the delivery of a severely premature infant.

Laura Wilson (Room 206)
37-week intrauterine pregnancy—A teenage Caucasian primigravida urgently admitted after being found unconscious. Her complications include HIV-positive status and chronic polysubstance abuse. Unrealistic expectations of parenthood and living with a chronic illness, combined with strained family relations, prompt comprehensive social and psychiatric evaluations initiated on the day of simulation.

PEDIATRIC UNIT

Tiffany Sheldon (Room 305)
Anorexia nervosa—A 14-year-old Caucasian female admitted for dehydration, electrolyte imbalance, and malnutrition following a syncope episode at home. This patient has a history of eating disorders that have required multiple hospital admissions and have strained family dynamics between mother and daughter.

SKILLED NURSING UNIT

Kathryn Doyle (Room 503)
Rehabilitation post left hip replacement—An elderly Caucasian female admitted following a complicated recovery from an ORIF. She is experiencing symptoms of malnutrition and depression due to unstable family dynamics, placing her at risk for elder abuse.

Carlos Reyes (Room 504)
Rehabilitation status post myocardial infarction—An elderly Hispanic male admitted for evaluation of the need for long-term care following an acute care hospital stay. Recent cognitive changes and a diagnosis of anxiety disorder contribute to stressful family dynamics and caregiver strain.

■ HOW TO SELECT A PATIENT

- You can choose one or more patients to work with from the Patient List by clicking the box to the left of the patient name(s). (In order to receive a scorecard for a patient, the patient must be selected before proceeding to the Nurses' Station.)
- Click on **Get Report** to the right of the medical records number (MRN) to view a summary of the patient's care during the 12-hour period before your arrival on the unit.
- After reviewing the report, click on **Return to Patient List**.
- When you are ready to begin your care, click on **Go to Nurses' Station** in the right lower corner.

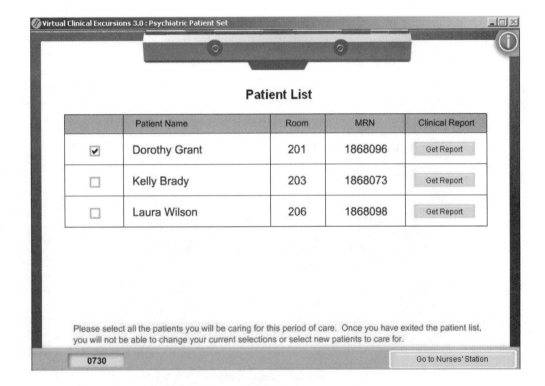

■ HOW TO FIND A PATIENT'S RECORDS

NURSES' STATION

Within the Nurses' Station, you will see:

1. A clipboard that contains the patient list for that floor.
2. A chart rack with patient charts labeled by room number, a notebook labeled Kardex, and a notebook labeled MAR (Medication Administration Record).
3. A desktop computer with access to the Electronic Patient Record (EPR).
4. A tool bar across the top of the screen that can also be used to access the Patient List, EPR, Chart, MAR, and Kardex. This tool bar is also accessible from each patient's room.
5. A Drug Guide containing information about the medications you are able to administer to your patients.

As you run your cursor over an item, it will be highlighted. To select, simply double-click on the item. As you use these resources, you will always be able to return to the Nurses' Station by clicking on the **Return to Nurses' Station** bar located in the right lower corner of your screen.

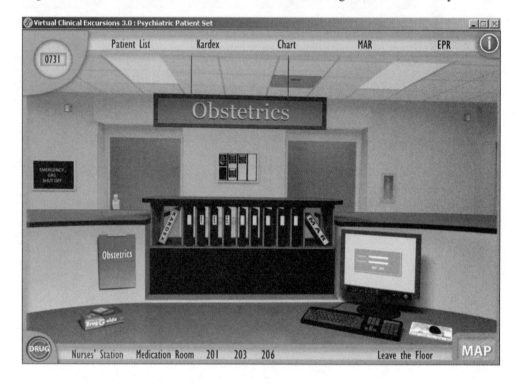

MEDICATION ADMINISTRATION RECORD (MAR)

The MAR icon located in the tool bar at the top of your screen accesses current 24-hour medications for each patient. Click on the icon and the MAR will open. (*Note:* You can also access the MAR by clicking on the blue MAR notebook on the far right side of the book rack in the center of the screen.) Within the MAR, tabs on the right side of the screen allow you to select patients by room number. Be careful to make sure you select the correct tab number for *your* patient rather than simply reading the first record that appears after the MAR opens. Each MAR sheet lists the following:

- Medications
- Route and dosage of medications
- Times of administration of medication

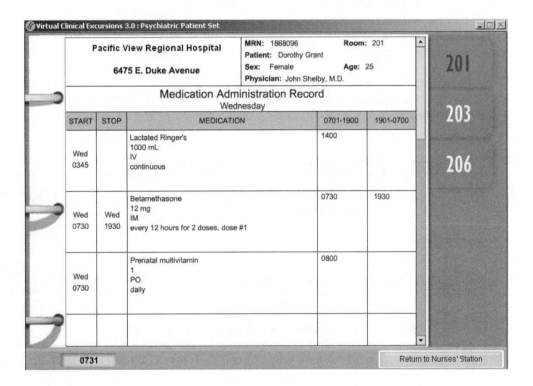

Note: The MAR changes each day. Expired MARs are stored in the patients' charts.

CHARTS

To access patient charts, either click on the **Chart** icon at the top of your screen or anywhere within the chart rack in the center of the Nurses' Station screen. When the close-up view appears, the individual charts are labeled by room number. To open a chart, click on the room number of the patient whose chart you wish to review. The patient's name and allergies will appear, along with a list of tabs on the right side of the screen, allowing you to view the following data:

- Allergies
- Physician's Orders
- Physician's Notes
- Nurse's Notes
- Laboratory Reports
- Diagnostic Reports
- Surgical Reports
- Consultations

- Patient Education
- History and Physical
- Nursing Admission
- Expired MARs
- Consents
- Mental Health
- Admissions
- Emergency Department

Information appears in real time. The entries are in reverse chronological order, so use the down arrow at the right side of the chart page to scroll down to view previous entries. Flip from tab to tab to view multiple data fields or click on the **Return to Nurses' Station** bar in the lower right corner of the screen to exit the chart.

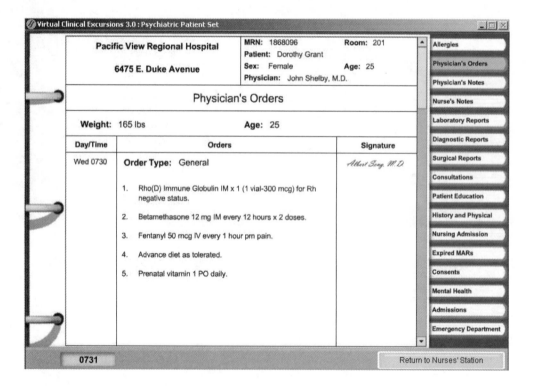

ELECTRONIC PATIENT RECORD (EPR)

The EPR can be accessed from the computer in the Nurses' Station or from the EPR icon located in the tool bar at the top of your screen. To access a patient's EPR:
- Click on either the computer screen or the **EPR** icon.
- Your user name and password are automatically filled in.
- Click on **Login** to enter the EPR.

The EPR used in Pacific View Regional Hospital represents a composite of commercial versions being used in hospitals. You can access the EPR:
- for a patient (by room number).
- to review existing data.
- to enter data you collect while working with a patient.

The EPR is updated daily, so no matter what day or part of a shift you are working, there will be a current EPR with the patient's data from the past days of the current hospital stay. This type of simulated EPR allows you to examine how data for different attributes have changed over time, as well as to examine data for all of a patient's attributes at a particular time. The EPR is fully functional (as it is in a real-life hospital). You can enter such data as blood pressure, breath sounds, and certain treatments. The EPR will not, however, allow you to enter data for a previous time period. Use the arrows at the bottom of the screen to move forward and backward in time.

Virtual Clinical Excursions 3.0 : Psychiatric Patient Set				0732
Patient: 201 Category: Vital Signs				
Name: Dorothy Grant	Wed 0345	Wed 0400	Wed 0500	Code Meanings
PAIN: LOCATION	A	A	A	A Abdomen
PAIN: RATING	1	1	2-3	Ar Arm
PAIN: CHARACTERISTICS	A	D	I	B Back
PAIN: VOCAL CUES		NN	NN	C Chest
PAIN: FACIAL CUES			FC2	Ft Foot
PAIN: BODILY CUES				H Head
PAIN: SYSTEM CUES	NN			Hd Hand
PAIN: FUNCTIONAL EFFECTS				L Left
PAIN: PREDISPOSING FACTORS		NN	NN	Lg Leg
PAIN: RELIEVING FACTORS		NN	NN	Lw Lower
PCA				N Neck
TEMPERATURE (F)		97.6		NN See Nurses notes
TEMPERATURE (C)				OS Operative site
MODE OF MEASUREMENT		O		Or See Physicians orders
SYSTOLIC PRESSURE		126		PN See Progress notes
DIASTOLIC PRESSURE		66		R Right
BP MODE OF MEASUREMENT		NIBP		Up Upper
HEART RATE		72		
RESPIRATORY RATE		18		
SpO2 (%)				
BLOOD GLUCOSE				
WEIGHT				
HEIGHT				

At the top of the EPR screen, you can choose patients by their room numbers. In addition, you have access to 17 different categories of patient data. To change patients or data categories, click the down arrow to the right of the room number or category.

The categories of patient data in the EPR as as follows:

- Vital Signs
- Respiratory
- Cardiovascular
- Neurologic
- Gastrointestinal
- Excretory
- Musculoskeletal
- Integumentary
- Reproductive
- Psychosocial
- Wounds and Drains
- Activity
- Hygiene and Comfort
- Safety
- Nutrition
- IV
- Intake and Output

Remember, each hospital selects its own codes. The codes used in the EPR at Pacific View Regional Hospital may be different from ones you have seen in clinical rotations that have computerized patient records. Take some time to acquaint yourself with the codes. Within the Vital Signs category, click on any item in the left column (e.g., heart rate). In the far-right column, you will see a list of code meanings for the possible findings and/or descriptors for that assessment area.

You will use the codes to record the data you collect as you work with patients. Click on the box in the last time column to the right of the data and wait for the code meanings applicable to that entry to appear. Select the appropriate code to describe your assessment findings and type it in the box. (*Note:* If no cursor appears within the box, click on the box again until the blue shading disappears and the blinking cursor appears.) Once the data are typed in this box, they are entered into the patient's record for this period of care only.

To leave the EPR, click on **Exit EPR** in the bottom right corner of the screen.

■ VISITING A PATIENT

From the Nurses' Station, click on the room number of the patient you wish to visit in the tool bar at the bottom of your screen. Once you are inside the room, you will see a still photo of your patient in the top left corner. To verify that this is the patient you have chosen, click on the **Check Armband** icon to the right of the photo. The patient's identification data will appear. If you click on **Check Allergies** (the next icon to the right), a list of the patient's allergies (if any) will replace the photo.

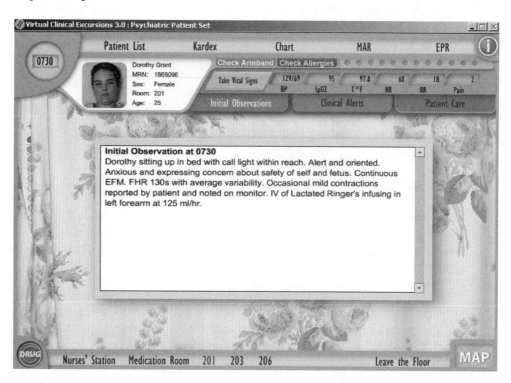

Also located in the patient's room are multiple icons you may use to assess the patient or the patient's medications. A clock is provided in the upper left corner of the room to monitor your progress in real time.

- The tool bar across the top of the screen allows you to check the **Patient List**, access the **EPR** to check or enter data, and view the patient's **Chart**, **MAR**, or **Kardex**.

- The **Take Vital Signs** icon allows you to measure the patient's up-to-the-minute blood pressure, oxygen saturation, temperature, heart rate, respiratory rate, and pain level.

- When you click on **Initial Observations**, a description appears in the text box under the patient's photo, allowing you a "look" at the patient as if you had just stepped in. To the right of this icon is **Clinical Alerts**, a resource that allows you to make decisions about priority medication interventions based on emerging data collected in real time. Check this screen throughout your period of care to avoid missing critical information related to recently ordered or STAT medications.

- Clicking on the **Patient Care** icon opens up three specific learning environments within the patient room: **Physical Assessment**, **Nurse-Client Interactions**, and **Medication Administration**.

- To perform a **Physical Assessment**, choose a body area (such as **Head & Neck**) by clicking on the appropriate icon in the column of yellow buttons. This activates a list of system subcategories for that body area (e.g., see **Sensory**, **Neurologic**, etc. in the green boxes). After you click on the system that you wish to evaluate, a still photo and text box appear, describing the assessment findings. The still photo is a "snapshot" of how an assessment of this area might be done or what the finding might look like. For every body area, there is also an **Equipment** button located on the far right of the screen.

- To the right of the Physical Assessment icon is **Nurse-Client Interactions**. Clicking on this icon will reveal the times and titles of any videos available for viewing. (*Note:* If the video you wish to see is not listed, this means you have not yet reached the correct virtual time to view that video. Check the virtual clock; you may return to access the video once its designated time has occurred—as long as you do so within the corresponding period of care.) To view a listed video, click on the white arrow to the right of the video title. Use the square control buttons below the video to start, stop, pause, rewind, or fast-forward the action or to mute the sound.

- **Medication Administration** is the pathway that allows you to review and administer medications to a patient after you have prepared them in the Medication Room. This process is addressed further in the *How to Prepare Medications* section (pages 19-20) and in *A Detailed Tour* (pages 26-30).

■ HOW TO QUIT, CHANGE PATIENTS, OR CHANGE PERIOD OF CARE

How to Quit: From most screens, you may click the **Leave the Floor** icon on the bottom tool bar to the right of the patient room numbers. (*Note:* From some screens, you will first need to click an **Exit** button or **Return to Nurses' Station** before clicking **Leave the Floor**.) When the Floor Menu appears, click **Exit** to leave the program.

How to Change Patients, Floors, or Period of Care: To change patients, simply click on the new patient's room number. (You cannot receive a scorecard for a new patient, however, unless you have already selected that patient on the Patient List screen.) To change to a new period of care, to change floors, or to restart the virtual clock for a new patient, click the **Leave the Floor** icon and then **Restart**.

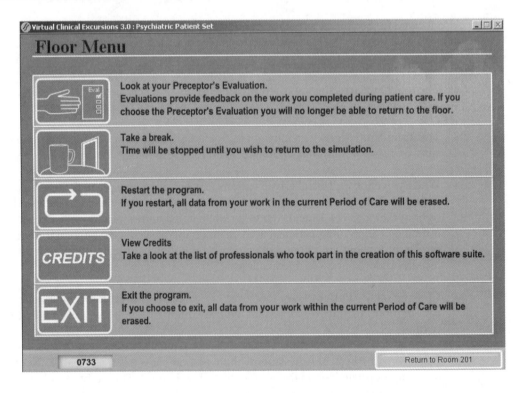

■ HOW TO PREPARE MEDICATIONS

From the Nurses' Station or the patient's room, you can access the Medication Room by clicking on the icon in the tool bar at the bottom of your screen to the left of the patient room numbers.

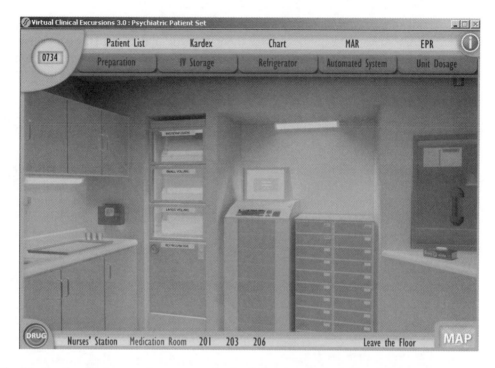

In the Medication Room you have access to the following (from left to right):

- A preparation area is located on the counter under the cabinets. To begin the medication preparation process, click on the tray on the counter or click on the **Preparation** icon at the top of the screen. The next screen leads you through a preparation sequence (called the Preparation Wizard) to prepare medications one at a time for administration to a patient. However, no medication has been selected at this time. We will do this while working with a patient in *A Detailed Tour*. To exit this screen, click on **View the Medication Room**.

- To the right of the cabinets (and above the refrigerator), IV storage bins are provided. Click on the bins themselves or on the **IV Storage** icon at the top of the screen. The bins are labeled **Microinfusion**, **Small Volume**, and **Large Volume**. Click on an individual bin to see a list of its contents. No medications are available in the bins at this time, but if they were, you could click on an individual medication and its label would appear to the right under the patient's name. Next, you would click **Put Medication on Tray**. If you ever change your mind or choose the incorrect medication, you can reverse your actions by clicking on **Put Medication in Bin**. Click **Close Bin** in the right bottom corner to exit. **View Medication Room** brings you back to a full view of the entire room.

- A refrigerator is located under the IV storage bins to hold any medications that must be stored below room temperature. Click on it to remove your medications; then click **Close Door**. You can also access this area by clicking the **Refrigerator** icon at the top of the screen.

- To prepare controlled substances, click the **Automated System** icon at the top of the screen or click the computer monitor located to the right of the IV storage bins. A login screen will appear; your name and password are automatically filled in. Click **Login**. Select a patient to log medications out for; then select the drawer you wish to open. Click **Open Drawer**, choose **Put Medication on Tray**, and then click **Close Drawer**.

- Next to the Automated System is a set of drawers identified by patient room number. To access these, click on the drawers themselves or on the **Unit Dosage** icon at the top of the screen. This provides a close-up view of the drawers. Click on the room number of the patient you are working with to open that drawer. Next, click on the medication you would like to prepare for the patient, and a label appears to the right under the patient's name, listing strength, units, and dosage per unit. You can **Open** and **Close** this medication label by clicking the appropriate icon. To exit, click **Close Drawer**; then click **View Medication Room**.

At any time, you can learn about a medication you wish to prepare for a patient by clicking on the **Drug** icon in the bottom left corner of the medication room screen or by clicking the **Drug Guide** book on the counter to the right of the unit dosage drawers. The **Drug Guide** provides information about the medications commonly included in nursing drug handbooks. Nutritional supplements and maintenance intravenous fluid preparations are not included.

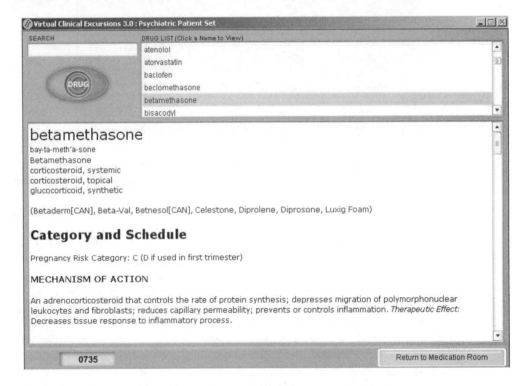

To access the MAR to review the medications ordered for a patient, click on the **MAR** icon located in the tool bar at the top of your screen. You may also click the **Review MAR** icon in the tool bar at the bottom of your screen from inside each medication storage area.

After you have chosen and prepared your medications, return to the patient's room to administer them by clicking on the room number in the bottom tool bar. Once inside the patient's room, click on **Medication Administration** and follow the administration sequence.

■ PRECEPTOR'S EVALUATIONS

When you have finished a session, click on **Leave the Floor** to go to the Floor Menu. At this point, you can click on the icon next to **Look at Your Preceptor's Evaluation** to receive a scorecard that provides feedback on the work you completed during patient care.

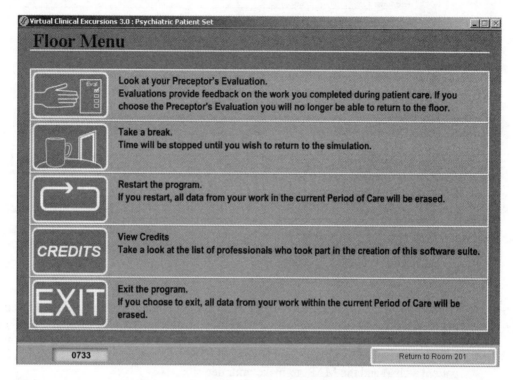

Evaluations are available for each patient you signed in for. Click on any of the **Medication Scorecard** icons to see an example. The scorecard compares the medications you administered to a patient during a period of care with what should have been administered. Table A lists the correct medications. Table B lists any medications that were administered incorrectly.

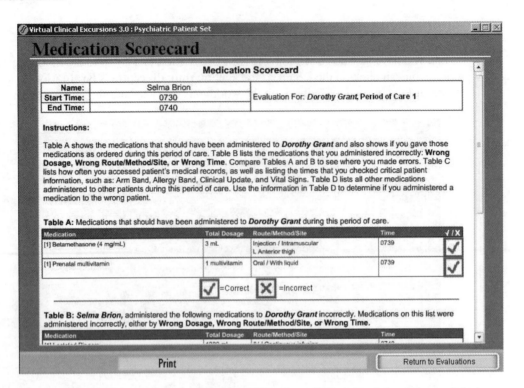

Not every medication listed on the MAR should be given. For example, a patient might have an allergy to a drug that was ordered, or a medication might have been improperly transcribed to the MAR. Predetermined medication "errors" embedded within the program challenge you to exercise critical thinking skills and professional judgment when deciding to administer a medication, just as you would in a real hospital. Use all your available resources, such as the patient's chart and the MAR, to make your decision.

Table C lists the resources that were available to assist you in medication administration, and it documents whether and when you accessed these resources. For example, did you check the patient armband or perform a check of vital signs? If so, when?

You can click **Print** to get a copy of this report if needed. Click **Return to Evaluations** when finished.

■ **FLOOR MAP**

To get a general sense of your location within the hospital, click on the **Map** icon found in the lower right corner of most of the screens in the *Virtual Clinical Excursions—Psychiatric* program. A floor map will appear, showing the layout of the floor you are currently on, as well as a directory of the patients and services on that floor. As you move your cursor over the directory list, the location of each room is highlighted (and vice versa). The floor map can be accessed from the Nurses' Station, Medication Room, and each patient's room.

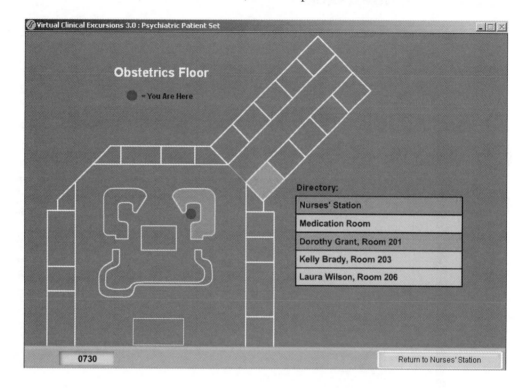

A DETAILED TOUR

If you wish to more thoroughly understand the capabilities of *Virtual Clinical Excursions—Psychiatric*, take a detailed tour by completing the following section. During this tour, we will work with a specific patient to introduce you to all the different components and learning opportunities available within the software.

■ WORKING WITH A PATIENT

Sign in and select the Obstetrics Floor for Period of Care 1 (0730-0815). From the Patient List, select Dorothy Grant in Room 201; however, do not go to the Nurses' Station yet.

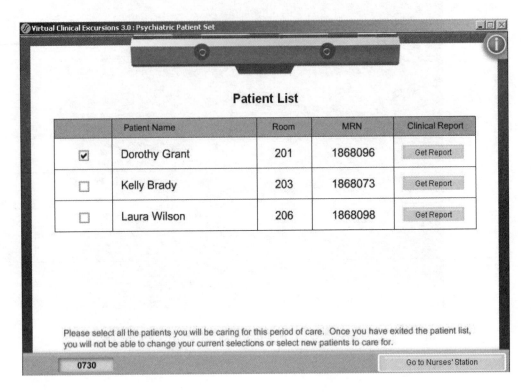

■ REPORT

In hospitals, when one shift ends and another begins, the outgoing nurse who attended a patient will give a verbal and sometimes a written summary of that patient's condition to the incoming nurse who will assume care for the patient. This summary is called a report and is an important source of data to provide an overview of a patient. Your first task is to get clinical report on Dorothy Grant. To do this, click **Get Report** in the far right column in this patient's row. From this summary, identify the problems and areas of concern that you will need to address for this patient.

When you have finished reading the report and noting any areas of concern, click on **Return to Patient List** and then on **Go to Nurses' Station**.

■ CHARTS

You can access Dorothy Grant's chart from the Nurses' Station or from the patient's room (201). We will access it from the Nurses' Station: Click on the chart rack or on the **Chart** icon in the tool bar at the top of your screen. Next, click on the chart labeled **201** to open the medical record for Dorothy Grant. Click on the **Emergency Department** tab to view a record of why this patient was admitted.

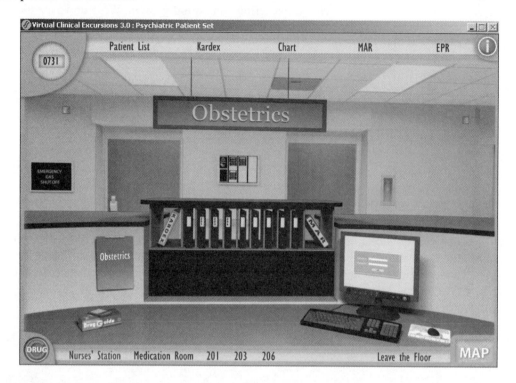

How many days has Dorothy Grant been in the hospital?

What tests were done upon her arrival in the Emergency Department and why?

What was her reason for admission?

You should also click on **Surgical Reports** to learn what procedures were performed and when. Finally, review the **Nursing Admission** and **History and Physical** tabs to view information on the health history of this patient. When you are done reviewing the chart, click **Return to Nurses' Station**.

■ MEDICATIONS

Open the Medication Administration Record (MAR) by clicking on the **MAR** icon in the tool bar at the top of your screen. *Remember:* The MAR automatically opens to the first occupied room number on the floor. Since you need to access Dorothy Grant's MAR, click on tab **201** (her room number). Always make sure you are giving the *Right Drug to the Right Patient!*

Examine the list of medications prescribed for Dorothy Grant. Write down the medications that need to be given during this period of care (0730-0815). For each medication, note the dosage, route, and time in the chart below.

Time	Medication	Dosage	Route

Click on **Return to Nurses' Station**. Next, click on **201** on the bottom tool bar and then verify that you are indeed in Dorothy Grant's room. Select **Clinical Alerts** (the icon to the right of Initial Observations) to check for any emerging data that might affect your medication administration priorities. Go to the patient's chart (click on the **Chart** icon; then click on **201**). When the chart opens, select the **Physician's Orders** tab.

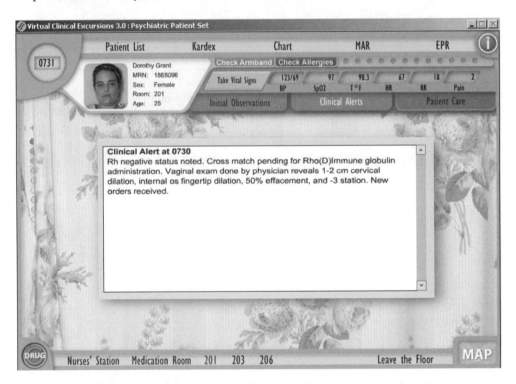

Review the orders. Have any new medications been ordered? Return to the MAR (click **Return to Room 201**; then click **MAR**). Verify that the new medications have been correctly transcribed to the MAR. Mistakes are sometimes made in the transcription process in the hospital setting, and it is sound practice to double-check any new order.

Are there any patient assessments you will need to perform before administering these medications? If so, return to Room 201 and click on **Review of Systems** to complete those before proceeding. (*Hint:* Check apical pulse.)

Now click on the **Medication Room** icon in the tool bar at the bottom of your screen to locate and prepare the medications for Dorothy Grant.

In the Medication Room, you must access the medications for Dorothy Grant from the specific dispensing system in which each medication is stored. Locate each medication that needs to be given in this time period and click on **Put Medication on Tray** as appropriate. (*Hint:* Look in Unit Dosage drawer first.) When you are finished, click on **Close Drawer** and then on **View Medication Room**. Now click on the medication tray on the counter on the left side of the medication room screen to begin preparing the medications you have selected. (*Note:* Instead of clicking on the tray, you can click **Preparation** at top of screen.)

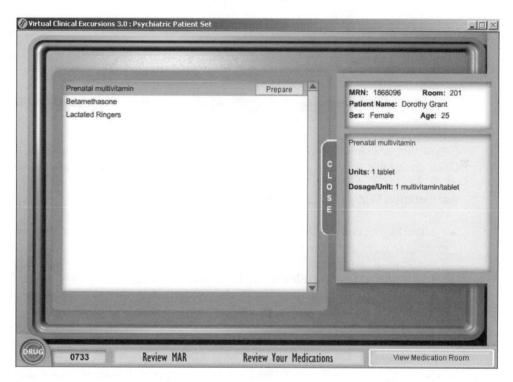

In the preparation area, you should see a list of the medications you put on the tray in the previous steps. Click on the first medication and then click **Prepare**. Follow the onscreen instructions of the Preparation Wizard, providing any data requested. As an example, let's follow the preparation process for betamethasone, one of the medications due to be administered to Dorothy Grant during this period of care. To begin, click to select **Betamethasone**; then click **Prepare**. Now work through the Preparation Wizard sequence as detailed below:

    Amount of medication in the ampule: Betamethasone 5 mL
    Enter the amount of medication you will draw up into a syringe: **3 mL**
    Click **Next**.
    Select the patient you wish to set aside the medication for:
    Click **Room 201, Dorothy Grant**.
    Click **Finish**.
    Click **Return to Medication Room**.

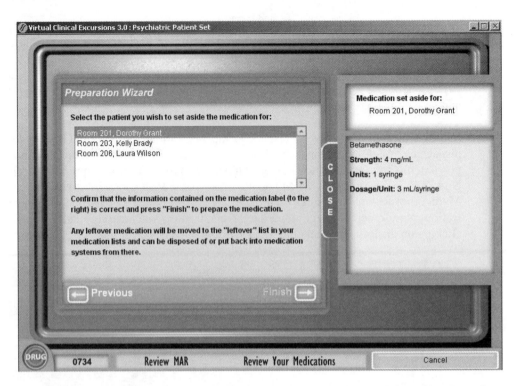

Follow this same basic process for the other medications due to be administered to Dorothy Grant during this period of care. (*Hint:* Look in **IV Storage** and **Automated System**.)

PREPARATION WIZARD EXCEPTIONS

- Some medications in *Virtual Clinical Excursions—Psychiatric* are preprepared by the pharmacy (e.g., IV antibiotics) and taken to the patient room as a whole. This is common practice in most hospitals.
- Blood products are not administered by students through the *Virtual Clinical Excursions—Psychiatric* simulations since blood administration follows specific protocols not covered in this program.
- The *Virtual Clinical Excursions—Psychiatric* simulations do not allow for mixing more than one type of medication, such as regular and Lente insulins, in the same syringe. In the clinical setting, when multiple types of insulin are ordered for a patient, the regular insulin is drawn up first, followed by the longer-acting insulin. Insulin is always administered in a special unit-marked syringe.

Now return to Room 201 (click on **201** on bottom tool bar) to administer Dorothy Grant's medications.

At any time during the medication administration process, you can perform a further review of systems, take vital signs, check information contained within the chart, or verify patient identity and allergies. Inside Dorothy Grant's room, click **Take Vital Signs**. (*Note:* These findings change over time to reflect the temporal changes you would find in a patient similar to Dorothy Grant.)

When you have gathered all the data you need, click on **Patient Care** and then select **Medication Administration**. After reviewing your medications, continue the administration process with the betamethasone ordered for Dorothy Grant. In the list of medications set aside for this patient, find **Betamethasone**. Next, click on the down arrow to the right of **Select** and choose **Administer** from the drop-down menu. This will activate the Administration Wizard. Complete the Wizard sequence as follows:

- Route: **Injection**
- Method: **Intramuscular**
- Site: **Any** (choose one)
- Click **Administer to Patient** arrow.
- Would you like to document this administration in the MAR? **Yes**
- Click **Finish** arrow.

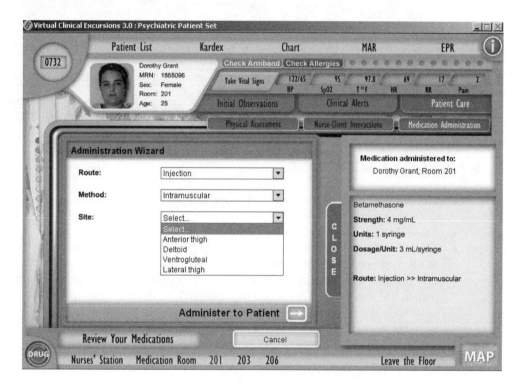

Selections are recorded by a tracking system and evaluated on a Medication Scorecard stored under Preceptor's Evaluations. This scorecard can be viewed, printed, and given to your instructor. To access the Preceptor's Evaluations, click on **Leave the Floor**. When the Floor Menu appears, click on the icon next to **Look at Your Preceptor's Evaluation**. From the list of evaluations, click on **Medication Scorecard** inside the box with Dorothy Grant's name.

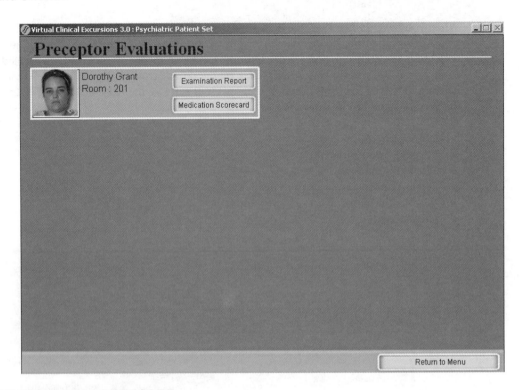

■ MEDICATION SCORECARD

- First, review Table A. Was betamethasone given correctly? Did you give the other medications as ordered?
- Table B shows you which (if any) medications you gave incorrectly.
- Table C addresses the resources used for Dorothy Grant. Did you access the patient's chart, MAR, EPR, or Kardex as needed to make safe medication administration decisions?
- Did you check the patient's armband to verify her identity? Did you check whether your patient had any known allergies to medications? Were vital signs taken?

■ VITAL SIGNS

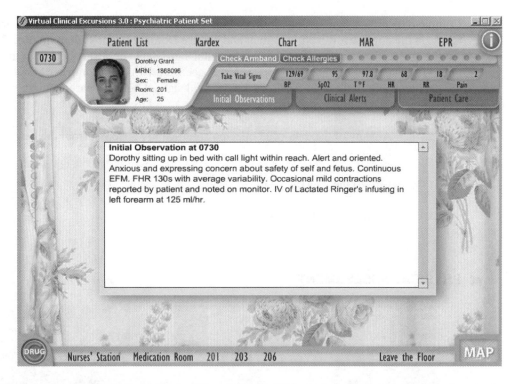

Vital signs, often considered the traditional signs of life, include body temperature, heart rate, respiratory rate, blood pressure, oxygen saturation of the blood, and the patient's experience of pain.

Inside Dorothy Grant's room, click **Take Vital Signs**. (*Remember:* You can take vital signs at any time. The data change over time to reflect the temporal changes you would find in a patient similar to Dorothy Grant.) Collect vital signs for this patient and record them in the following table. Note the time at which you collected each of these data.

Vital Signs	Findings/Time
Blood pressure	
O$_2$ saturation	
Heart rate	
Respiratory rate	
Temperature	
Pain rating	

After you are done, click on the **EPR** icon located in the tool bar at the top of the screen.

Complete the EPR Login screen as directed in *A Quick Tour* (see page 15 of this workbook). Click on the down arrow next to Patient and choose Dorothy Grant's room number **201**. Select **Vital Signs** as the category. Next, record the vital signs data you just collected in the last column. (*Note:* If you need help with this process, see page 16.) Now compare these findings with the data you collected earlier for this patient's vital signs. Use these earlier findings to establish a baseline for each of the vital signs.

    a. Are any of the data you collected significantly different from the baseline for a particular vital sign?

        Circle One: Yes   No

    b. If "Yes," which data are different?

■ PHYSICAL ASSESSMENT

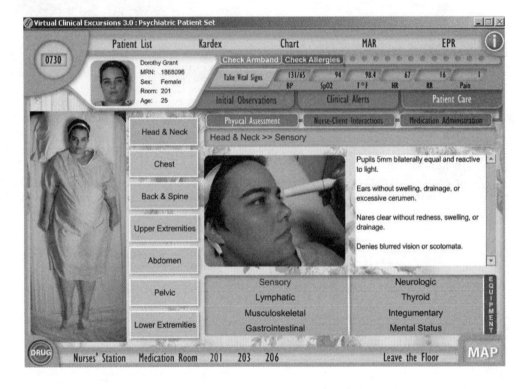

After you have finished examining the EPR for vital signs, click **Exit EPR** to return to Room 201. Click **Patient Care** and then **Physical Assessment**. Think about what information you received in report, as well as what you may have learned about this patient from the chart. What area(s) of examination should you pay most attention to at this time? Is there any equipment you should be monitoring? Conduct a physical assessment of the body areas and systems that you consider priorities for Dorothy Grant. For example, select **Head & Neck**; then click on and assess **Mental Status** and **Equipment**. Complete any other assessment(s) you think are necessary at this time. In the following table, record the data you collected during this examination.

Area of Examination	Findings
Head & Neck Mental Status	
Head & Neck Equipment	

After you have finished collecting these data, return to the EPR. Compare the data that were already in the record with those you just collected.

    a.   Are any of the data you collected significantly different from the baselines for this patient?

        Circle One: Yes   No

    b.   If "Yes," which data are different?

■ NURSE-CLIENT INTERACTIONS

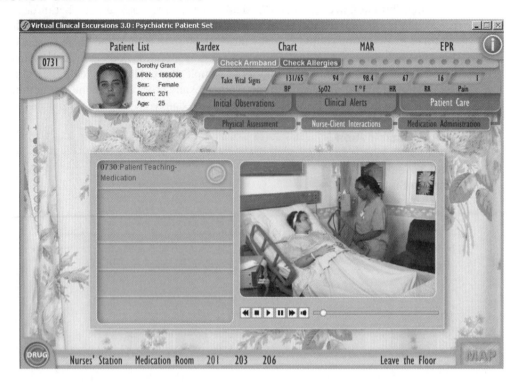

Click on **Patient Care** from inside Dorothy Grant's room (201). Now click on **Nurse-Client Interactions** to access a short video titled **Patient Teaching—Medication**, which is available for viewing at 0735 (based on the virtual clock in the upper left corner of your screen). To begin the video, click on the arrow next to its title. You will observe a nurse communicating with Dorothy Grant. There are many variations of nursing practice, some exemplifying "best" practice and some not. Note whether the nurse in this interaction displays professional behavior and compassionate care. Are her words congruent with what is going on with the patient? Does this interaction "feel right" to you? If not, how would you handle this situation differently? Explain.

Note: If the video you wish to view is not listed, this means you have not yet reached the correct virtual time to view that video. Check the virtual clock; you may return to access the video once its designated time has occurred—as long as you do so within the corresponding period of care.

At least one Nurse-Client Interactions video is available during each period of care. Viewing these videos can help you learn more about what is occurring with a patient at a certain time and also prompt you to discriminate between nurse communications that are ideal and those that need improvement. Compassionate care and the ability to communicate clearly are essential components of delivering quality nursing care, and it is during your clinical time that you will begin to refine these skills.

■ COLLECTING AND EVALUATING DATA

Each of the activities you perform in the Patient Care environment generates a great deal of assessment data. Remember that after you collect data, you can record your findings in the EPR. You can also review the EPR, patient's chart, videos, and MAR at any time. You will get plenty of practice collecting and then evaluating data in context of the patient's course.

Now, here's an important question for you:

> Did the previous sequence of exercises provide the most efficient way to assess Dorothy Grant?

For example, you went to the patient's room to get vital signs, then back to the EPR to enter data and compare your findings with extant data. Next, you went back to the patient's room to do a physical examination, then again back to the EPR to enter and review data. If this back-and-forth process of data collection and recording seemed inefficient, remember the following:

- Plan all of your nursing activities to maximize efficiency while at the same time optimizing quality of patient care. (Think about what data you might need to perform certain tasks. For example, do you need to check a heart rate before administering a cardiac medication or check an IV site before starting an infusion?)

- You collect a tremendous amount of data when you work with a patient. Very few people can accurately remember all these data for more than a few minutes. Develop efficient assessment skills, and record data as soon as possible after collecting them.

- Assessment data are only the starting point for the nursing process.

Make a clear distinction between these first exercises and how you actually provide nursing care. These initial exercises were designed to involve you actively in the use of different software components. This workbook focuses on sensible practices for implementing the nursing process in ways that ensure the highest quality care of patients.

Most important, remember that a human being changes through time, and that these changes include both the physical and psychosocial facets of a person as a living organism. Think about this for a moment. Some patients may change physically in a very short time (a patient with emerging myocardial infarction) or more slowly (a patient with a chronic illness). Patients' overall physical and psychosocial conditions may improve or deteriorate. They may have effective coping skills and familial support, or they may feel alone and full of despair. In fact, each individual is a complex mix of physical and psychosocial elements, and at least some of these elements usually change through time.

Thus it is crucial *not* to think of the nursing process as a simple one-time, five-step procedure:

- Assessment
- Nursing Diagnosis
- Planning
- Implementation
- Evaluation

Rather, the nursing process should be utilized as a creative and systematic approach to delivering nursing care. Furthermore, because all living organisms are constantly changing, we must apply the nursing process over and over. Each time we follow the nursing process for an individual patient, we refine our understanding of that patient's physical and psychosocial conditions based on collection and analysis of many different types of data. *Virtual Clinical Excursions—Psychiatric* will help you develop both the creativity and the systematic approach needed to become a nurse who is equipped to deliver the highest quality care to all patients.

■ **REDUCING MEDICATION ERRORS: SELF-EVALUATION**

Earlier in this detailed tour, you learned the basic steps of medication preparation and administration. The following simulations will allow you to practice those skills further—with an increased emphasis on reducing medication errors by using the Medication Scorecard to evaluate your work.

Sign in to work at Pacific View Regional Hospital for Period of Care 1. (*Note:* If you are already working with another patient or during another period of care, click on **Leave the Floor** and then **Restart the Program**; then sign in.)

From the Patient List, select Dorothy Grant. Then click on **Go To Nurses' Station**. Complete the following steps to prepare and administer medications to Dorothy Grant.

- Click on **Medication Room**.
- Click on **MAR** to determine prn medications that have been ordered for Dorothy Grant to address his constipation and pain. (*Note:* You may click on **Review MAR** at any time to verify correct medication order. Remember to look at the patient name on the MAR to make sure you have the correct patient's record—you must click on the correct room number within the MAR.) Click on **Return to Medication Room** after reviewing the correct MAR.
- Click on **Unit Dosage** (or on the Unit Dosage cabinet); from the close-up view, click on drawer **201**.
- Select the medications you would like to administer. After each selection, click **Put Medication on Tray**. When you are finished selecting medications, click **Close Drawer**.
- Click on **View Medication Room**.
- Click on **Automated System** (or on the Automated System unit itself). Click **Login**.
- On the next screen, specify the correct patient and drawer location.
- Select the medication you would like to administer and click on **Put Medication on Tray**. Repeat this process if you wish to administer other medications from the Automated System.
- When you are finished, click **Close Drawer**. At the bottom right corner of the next screen, click on **View Medication Room**.
- From the Medication Room, click on **Preparation** (or on the preparation tray).
- From the list of medications on your tray, choose the correct medication to administer.
- Click **Next**, specify the correct patient to administer this medication to, and click **Finish**.
- Repeat the previous two steps until all medications that you want to administer are prepared.
- You can click on **Review Your Medications** and then on **Return to Medication Room** when ready. Once you are back in the Medication Room, go directly to Dorothy Grant's room by clicking on **201** at bottom of screen.
- Inside the patient's room, administer the medication, utilizing the five rights of medication administration. After you have collected the appropriate assessment data and are ready for administration, click **Patient Care** and then **Medication Administration**. Verify that the correct patient and medication(s) appear in the left-hand window. Then click the down arrow next to Select. From the drop-down menu, select **Administer** and complete the Administration Wizard by providing any information requested. When the Wizard stops asking for information, click **Administer to Patient**. Specify **Yes** when asked whether this administration should be recorded in the MAR. Finally, click **Finish**.

Now let's see how you did during your earlier medication administration!

- Click on **Leave the Floor** at the bottom of your screen. From the Floor Menu, select **Look at Your Preceptor's Evaluation**. Then click on **Medication Scorecard**.

These resources will help you find out more about each patient's medications and possible sources of medication errors.

1. Start by examining Table A. These are the medications you should have given to Dorothy Grant during this period of care. If each of the medications in Table A has a √ by it, then you made no errors. Congratulations!

If there are some medications that have an X by them, then you made one or more medication errors.

Compare Tables A and B to determine which of the following types of errors you made: Wrong Dose, Wrong Route/Method/Site, or Wrong Time. Follow these steps:
   a. Find medications in Table A that were given incorrectly.
   b. Now see if those same medications are in Table B, which shows what you actually administered to Dorothy Grant.
   c. Comparing Tables A and B, match the Strength, Dose, Route/Method/Site, and Time for each medication you administered incorrectly.
   d. Then, using the form below, list the medications given incorrectly and mark the errors you made for each medication.

Medication	Strength	Dosage	Route	Method	Site	Time
	❑	❑	❑	❑	❑	❑
	❑	❑	❑	❑	❑	❑
	❑	❑	❑	❑	❑	❑
	❑	❑	❑	❑	❑	❑

2. To help you reduce future medication errors, consider the following list of possible reasons for errors.

   • Did not check drug against MAR for correct patient, correct date, correct time, correct drug, and correct dose.
   • Did not check drug dose against MAR three times.
   • Did not open the unit dose package in the patient's room.
   • Did not correctly identify the patient using two identifiers.
   • Did not administer the drug on time.
   • Did not verify patient allergies.
   • Did not check the patient's current condition or vital sign parameters.
   • Did not consider why the patient would be receiving this drug.
   • Did not question why the drug was in the patient's drawer.
   • Did not check the physician's order and/or check with the pharmacist when there was a question about the drug or dose.
   • Did not verify that no adverse effects had occurred from a previous dose.

Based on these possibilities, determine how you made each error and record the reason into the form below:

Medication	Reason for Error

3. Look again at Table B. Are there medications listed that are not in Table A? If so, you gave a medication to Dorothy Grant that he should not have received. Complete the following exercises to help you understand how such an error might have been made.

    a. Perhaps you gave a medication that was on Dorothy Grant's MAR for this period of care, without recognizing that a change had occurred in the patient's condition that should have caused you to reconsider. Review patient records as necessary and complete the following form:

Medication	Possible Reasons Not to Give This Medication

    b. Another possibility is that you gave Dorothy Grant a medication that should have been given at a different time. Check his MAR and complete the form below to determine whether you made a Wrong Time error:

Medication	Given to Dorothy Grant at What Time	Should Have Been Given at What Time

c. Maybe you gave another patient's medication to Dorothy Grant. In this case, you made a Wrong Patient error. Check the MARs of other patients and use the form below to determine whether you made this type of error:

Medication	Given to Dorothy Grant	Should Have Been Given to

4. The Medication Scorecard provides some other interesting sources of information. For example, if there is a medication selected for Dorothy Grant but it was not given to him, there will be an X by that medication in Table A, but it will not appear in Table B. In that case, you might have given this medication to some other patient, which is another type of Wrong Patient error. To investigate further, look at Table D, which lists the medications you gave to other patients. See whether you can find any medications for Dorothy Grant that were given to another patient by mistake. Before making any decisions, be sure to cross-check the other patients' MAR because they may have had the same medication ordered. Use the following form to record your findings:

Medication	Should Have Been Given to Dorothy Grant	Given by Mistake to

5. Now take some time to review the exercises you just completed. Use the form below to create an overall analysis of what you have learned. Once again, record each of the medication errors you made, including the type of each error. Then, for each error you made, indicate specifically what you would do differently to prevent this type of error from occurring again.

Medication	Type of Error	Error Prevention Tactic

Submit this form to your instructor if required as a graded assignment, or simply use these exercises to improve your understanding of medication errors and how to reduce them.

Name: _____   Date: _____

The following icons are used throughout the workbook to help you quickly identify particular activities and assignments:

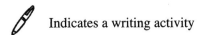 Indicates a reading assignment—tells you which textbook chapter(s) you should read before starting each lesson

Indicates a writing activity

Marks the beginning of an interactive CD-ROM activity—signals you to open or return to your *Virtual Clinical Excursions—Psychiatric* CD-ROM

Indicates additional CD-ROM instructions

Indicates questions and activities that require you to consult your textbook

Indicates the approximate time required to complete an exercise

LESSON 1

The Therapeutic Nurse-Patient Relationship

∽ **Reading Assignment:** Therapeutic Nurse-Patient Relationship (Chapter 2)

Patients: Jacquline Catanazaro, Medical-Surgical Floor, Room 402
Kathryn Doyle, Skilled Nursing Floor, Room 503

Goal: To demonstrate an understanding of the importance of the therapeutic nurse-patient relationship and be able to identify and use therapeutic communication techniques with patients.

Objectives:

- Understand the concept of the therapeutic nurse-patient relationship.
- Identify the personal qualities of the nurse that are necessary to communicate effectively.
- Define the phases of a therapeutic nurse-patient relationship.
- Observe and identify effective communication techniques used by the nurse in nurse-patient interactions.
- Discuss the concept of facilitative communication.
- Define and discuss the importance of the nurse possessing skills of genuineness, respect, and empathy in the therapeutic nurse-patient relationship.
- Understand types of therapeutic impasses and their relevance to the nurse-patient relationship.

 In this lesson you will learn the essential components of the therapeutic nurse-patient relationship. You will observe and record nurse-patient interactions to identify verbal and nonverbal techniques used in the nurse-patient interactions. Begin this activity by reviewing the therapeutic nurse-patient concepts in Chapter 2 in your textbook.

Exercise 1

 Clinical Preparation: Writing Activity

 30 minutes

1. Define the therapeutic nurse-patient relationship.

2. The key therapeutic tool of the psychiatric nurse is the _____.

3. There are six personal qualities the nurse must have in order to communicate

    therapeutically with patients. They are _____, _____,

    _____, _____,

    _____, and _____.

4. Discuss facilitative communication and its verbal and nonverbal components.

5. Discuss the qualities of genuineness, respect, and empathy that a nurse must have in order
   to establish and maintain a therapeutic relationship.

6. Define *therapeutic impasses* and discuss the four types of therapeutic impasses that can occur in a therapeutic relationship.

Exercise 2

 CD-ROM Activity

 30 minutes

- Sign in to work at Pacific View Regional Hospital on the Medical-Surgical Floor for Period of Care 1. (*Note:* If you are already in the virtual hospital from a previous exercise, click on **Leave the Floor** and then **Restart the Program** to get to the sign-in window.)
- Select Jacquline Catanazaro, Room 402.
- Click on **Get Report**.
- After reviewing the report, click on **Return to Patient List** and then on **Go to Nurses' Station**.
- Click on Room **402** at the bottom of the screen.
- Click on **Patient Care**.
- Click on **Nurse-Client Interactions**.
- Select and view the video titled: **0730: Intervention—Airway**. As you observe the nurse's verbal and nonverbal communication, complete the top row of the tables in questions 1 and 2.

Now let's jump ahead in virtual time to observe another interaction with this same patient.

- Click on **Leave the Floor**; then select **Restart the Program**.
- Sign in again for Jacquline Catanazaro on the Medical-Surgical Floor, but this time choose Period of Care 2.
- Click on **Go to Nurses' Station**.
- Click on **402** to return to the patient's room.
- Click on **Patient Care** and then on **Nurse-Client Interactions**.
- Select and view the video titled **1115: Assessment—Readiness to Learn**. As you watch and listen to the video, complete the middle row of the tables in questions 1 and 2.

Now let's see how a nurse communicates with an older patient on the Skilled Nursing Floor.

- First, **Leave the Floor** and **Restart the Program**.
- This time choose the Skilled Nursing Floor during Period of Care 1 and select Kathryn Doyle as your patient. Click on **Go to Nurses' Station**.
- Next, click on **503**, then on **Patient Care**, and then on **Nurse-Client Interactions**.
- Select and view the video titled: **0730: Assessment—Biopsychosocial**. Use this video interaction to complete the bottom row in the tables in questions 1 and 2.

 1. Based on the three videos you just viewed, complete the table below by listing the therapeutic verbal communications used by the nurses. For each technique you list, identify the specific nurse communication you observed that demonstrates the technique. (*Hint:* Consult pages 29-37 in your textbook.)

Patient/POC	Verbal Therapeutic Communication Techniques Used by Nurse	Nurse Communication That Demonstrates Technique
Jacquline Catanazaro POC 1		
Jacquline Catanazaro POC 2		
Kathryn Doyle POC 1		

2. Based on the same three videos you used for question 1, document the nurses' nonverbal therapeutic communication techniques in the table below.

Patient/POC	Nonverbal Communication	Nonverbal Therapeutic Techniques Used by the Nurse
Jacquline Catanazaro POC 1		
Jacquline Catanazaro POC 2		
Kathryn Doyle POC 1		

LESSON **2**

The Stuart Stress Adaptation Model of Psychiatric Nursing Care

Reading Assignment: The Stuart Stress Adaptation Model of Psychiatric Nursing Care (Chapter 4)

Patient: Kelly Brady, Obstetrics Floor, Room 203

Goal: To care for a patient with both medical and psychiatric illness utilizing the Stuart Stress Adaptation Model.

Objectives:

- Identify the biopsychosocial components of care using the Stress Adaptation Model.
- Use the Stress Adaptation Model to assess patients.
- Participate in the care of an obstetric patient who has a comorbid psychiatric disorder.
- Identify the predisposing and precipitating stressors of the identified patient.
- Evaluate the significance of the patient's stressors.
- Determine patient's coping resources and coping mechanisms.
- Identify the patient's stage of treatment and implement corresponding nursing interventions.

Exercise 1

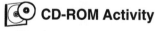 **CD-ROM Activity**

 45 minutes

- Sign in to work at Pacific View Regional Hospital on the Obstetrics Floor for Period of Care 3. (*Note:* If you are already in the virtual hospital from a previous exercise, click on **Leave the Floor** and then **Restart the Program** to get to the sign-in window.)
- Select Kelly Brady, Room 203.
- Click on **Get Report**. Review the report; then click on **Return to Patient List**.
- Click on **Go to Nurses' Station**.
- Click on **Chart** and then on **203**.
- Click on the **Nursing Admission**.

1. In the Nursing Admission, the aspect of Kelly Brady's history that indicates she has

   had mental health problems in the past is _____.

2. The three recent stressful life events that might contribute to Kelly Brady's depression and

   anxiety are _____

   _____.

3. How does Kelly Brady physically express her depression?
   a. Cries often and does not want to be alone
   b. Does not show her sadness
   c. Rocks back and forth
   d. Talks with friends

4. According to the Nursing Admission, what is Kelly Brady's main coping mechanism?

5. How does Kelly Brady feel about her hospitalization?

As you continue caring for Kelly Brady, use the information you have read in her chart and change-of-shift report and on pages 71-72 of your textbook.

→ • Click on **Return to Nurses' Station**.
   • Click on Room **203** at the bottom of the screen.
   • Click on **Patient Care**.
   • Click on **Nurse-Client Interactions**.
   • Select and view the video titled: **1500: Transfer to Labor and Delivery**. (*Note:* If this video is not available, check the virtual clock to see whether enough time has elapsed. The video cannot be viewed before its specified time.)

6. Considering the final aspect of the Stress Adaptation Model, what is Kelly Brady's treatment stage?
   a. Crisis
   b. Acute
   c. Maintenance
   d. Health Promotion

7. Given Kelly Brady's stage of treatment, complete the form below to identify the nurse's goal, assessment, interventions, and expected outcomes. For each of these components, identify the nurse's action within the video interaction that illustrates your answer.

a. What is the overall nursing goal?

   Nurse's action in video:

b. What should the nurse assessment focus on?

   Nurse's action in video:

c. What is the purpose of the nurse's intervention?

   Nurse's action in video:

d. What is the expected outcome?

   Nurse's action in video:

3 —————————————————————————

The Biopsychosocial, Cultural, and Spiritual Context of Nursing Care

——————————————————————————————————————

👓 **Reading Assignment:** Biological Context of Psychiatric Nursing Care (Chapter 6)
Psychological Context of Psychiatric Nursing Care (Chapter 7)
Social, Cultural, and Spiritual Context of Psychiatric Nursing
Care (Chapter 8)

Patient: Carlos Reyes, Skilled Nursing Floor, Room 504

Goal: To be able to discuss the biopsychosocial, cultural, and spiritual aspects of nursing care.

Objectives:

* Understand normal structure and function of the brain.
* Define neurotransmission as it relates to brain function and psychiatric disorders.
* Understand the function and content of the mental status examination to determine mental health functioning.
* Understand the role culture plays in the diagnosis and treatment of mental illness.
* Understand the risk factors associated with age, gender, education, and income in relation to mental health/illness.

Exercise 1

  CD-ROM Activity

🕒 45 minutes

* Sign in to work at Pacific View Regional Hospital on the Skilled Nursing Floor for Period of Care 1. (*Note:* If you are already in the virtual hospital from a previous exercise, click on **Leave the Floor** and then **Restart the Program** to get to the sign-in window.)
* Select Carlos Reyes, Room 504.
* Click on **Get Report**.
* Click on **Go to Nurses' Station**.
* Click on **Chart** and then on **504**.
* Read the **History and Physical** and **Nursing Admission** sections.

1. According to the History and Physical and the Nursing Admission, Carlos Reyes has two

   psychiatric diagnoses: _____ and _____.

2. Match each part of the brain to its function as it relates to Carlos Reyes' diagnoses.

Part of the Brain	**Function**
_____ Limbic system	a. Learning, abstracting, reasoning
_____ Temporal lobe	b. Attention, emotions, memory
_____ Frontal lobe	c. Verbal and speech behaviors

   - Click on **Return to Nurses' Station**.
   - Click on Room **504** at the bottom of the screen.
   - Click on **Patient Care**.
   - Click on **Physical Assessment**.
   - Next, select **Head & Neck**.
   - Then, click on **Mental Status**.

3. The mental status report reveals which of the following important information?
   a. Oriented to person and place only
   b. Sluggish speech patterns
   c. Impaired short-term memory
   d. High anxiety and agitation
   e. a, b, and c only

4. Two biological factors affecting Carlos Reyes' brain function that need to be considered in

   caring for him are _____ and _____.

5. Discuss the biopsychosocial and cultural factors that must be considered in caring for
   Carlos Reyes.

→ • Still in the patient's room, click on **Nurse-Client Interactions**.
  • Select and view the video titled **0740: Family Teaching—Medication**.
  • Now click on the **Drug** icon in the lower left corner. Using either the Search box or the scroll bar at the top of the screen, find the entry for oxazepam.

  6. Identify the indication(s) for oxazepam and the effect it has on brain function. What side effect was concerning Carlos Reyes' son during the video?

→ • Now, select and view the video titled **0745: Drowsiness—Contributing Factor**. (*Note:* If this video is not available, check the virtual clock to see whether enough time has elapsed. The video cannot be viewed before its specified time.)

  7. The two interventions the nurse used to answer Carlos Reyes' son's concerns regarding his

     father's drowsiness were _____ and

     _____.

  8.   What other actions could the nurse have taken?

→ • Finally, select and view the video titled **0750: Assessment—Level of Assistance**.

  9. What aspects of the mental status examination is the nurse attempting to assess?
     a. Appearance, speech, motor activity, and interaction
     b. Level of consciousness
     c. Emotional state: mood and affect
     d. All of the above

10. Assess the level of assistance Carlos Reyes will need in order to sit up and eat his breakfast.

LESSON 4

Family as Resources, Caregivers, and Collaborators

Reading Assignment: Families as Resources, Caregivers, and Collaborators
(Chapter 11)

Patient: Jacquline Catanazaro, Medical-Surgical Floor, Room 402

Goal: To understand the role of the family in caring for a patient with mental illness.

Objectives:

- Identify the characteristics of functional families.
- Learn the benefits of working with the families of patients with mental illness.
- Identify barriers involved in educating families.

Exercise 1

Clinical Preparation: Writing Activity

 30 minutes

1. The ten characteristics of a functional family are listed below and on the next page.
   Describe the qualities of each of these characteristics.

Characteristics of a Health Family	Qualities
1. Life cycle tasks	
2. Handling conflict	
3. Emotional contact	

Characteristics of a Health Family	Qualities
4. Boundaries	
5. Problem solving	
6. Differences	
7. Children	
8. Emotional climate	
9. Balance	
10. Communication	

2. Partnering with _____ is an essential part of nursing care.

3. List at least two benefits of working with the families of patients with mental illness.

4. Describe a best practice intervention that is helpful to families of patients with mental illness.

5. List four barriers the nurse might experience in working with families.

Exercise 2

  CD-ROM Activity

30 minutes

- Sign in to work at Pacific View Regional Hospital on the Medical-Surgical Floor for Period of Care 2. (*Note:* If you are already in the virtual hospital from a previous exercise, click on **Leave the Floor** and then **Restart the Program** to get to the sign-in window.)
- Select Jacquline Catanazaro in Room 402.
- Click on **Go to Nurses' Station**.
- Click on **Chart** and then on **402**.
- Review the **Nursing Admission** and **History and Physical** sections.

1. What family information would you consider helpful to know before working with Jacquline Catanazaro's family?

2. A complete family history usually includes:
   a. information about all family members across three generations.
   b. the use of a genogram to organize the information.
   c. the health status of all members.
   d. current household living arrangements.
   e. relationships among the members.
   f. all of the above.

3. Discuss why you think it is important for the nurse to provide patient teaching regarding Jacquline Catanazaro's medication with her sister present?

4. What are two issues the sister will most likely have to deal with after Jacquline Catanazaro is discharged?

5. The type of family education program that would be most helpful to Jacquline Catanazaro's sister would include:
   a. education about mental illness and community resources.
   b. practical approaches to help them cope with symptomatic behavior.
   c. reinforcing of family strengths.
   d. allowing family members to share their concerns.
   e. all of the above.

LESSON 5 _____

Crisis Intervention

_____

👓 **Reading Assignment:** Crisis Intervention (Chapter 14)

Patient: Dorothy Grant, Obstetrics Floor, Room 201

Goal: To understand how to provide nursing care for a patient in a health crisis using crisis intervention theory and techniques.

Objectives:

- Define the characteristics and types of crises.
- Describe the phases of a response to a crisis.
- Understand two types of crises.
- Define crisis and crisis intervention.
- Discuss the cultural factors related to crisis intervention.
- Understand the steps in crisis intervention.
- Knowledge of techniques used to deal with patients in crisis.

In this lesson, you will learn to identify a patient in crisis, understand the characteristics of and patient responses to the crisis, and take steps to help your patient deal with the crisis using crisis intervention theory and techniques.

Begin this lesson by reviewing the key concepts presented in your textbook. Answer the following questions to reinforce your understanding of the concepts.

Exercise 1

Clinical Preparation: Writing Activity

🕐 30 minutes

1. A _____ is a disturbance caused by a stressful event or a perceived threat.

2. Describe four phases in a response to a crisis.

3. The three balancing factors in a crisis that help an individual see the crisis realistically, support the individual in solving the problem, and offer effective coping are

   _____, _____, and

   _____.

4. Describe two types of crises and give an example of each.

5. _____ is a brief, focused, and time-limited (approximately 6 weeks in length) treatment strategy that has been shown to be effective in helping people effectively cope with stressful events in their lives. The goal of crisis intervention is to help

   the individual _____.

6. Describe how culture can play a crucial role in crisis intervention.

7. Explain the steps the nurse would take in providing crisis intervention and list the corresponding crisis intervention components within the step.

Crisis Intervention Steps	Crisis Intervention Components
Assessment	
Planning and implementation	
Evaluation	

 8. Match each crisis intervention technique to its definition. (*Hint:* See Box 14-2 in your textbook.)

Technique	Definition
_____ Catharsis	a. Nurse helps the patient to regain feelings of self-worth
_____ Clarification	b. Nurse reinforces healthy behavior
_____ Suggestion	c. Nurse promotes the release of feelings by the patient
_____ Reinforcement of behavior	d. Nurse and patient actively explore solutions to the crisis
_____ Support of defenses	e. Nurse helps the patient identify the relationship between the events, behaviors, and feelings
_____ Raising self-esteem	f. Nurse encourages the use of healthy defenses and discourages those that are maladaptive
_____ Exploration of solutions	g. Nurse influences the patient to accept an idea or belief

Exercise 2

  CD-ROM Activity

 30 minutes

- Sign in to work at Pacific View Regional Hospital on the Obstetrics Floor for Period of Care 1. (*Note:* If you are already in the virtual hospital from a previous exercise, click on **Leave the Floor** and then **Restart the Program** to get to the sign-in window.)
- Select Dorothy Grant in Room 201.
- Click on **Get Report**.

1. What information in the shift report would alert the nurse that a more thorough psychosocial assessment is needed?

It is important for the nurse to obtain more complete information in caring for Dorothy Grant.

→ - First, click on **Return to Patient List**.
- Now click on **Go to Nurses' Station**.
- Click on **Chart** and then on **201**.
- Access and review the **History and Physical** and **Nursing Admission** sections.

2. In the History and Physical, what information indicates that Dorothy Grant may be in crisis?
   a. Dorothy Grant is 30 weeks pregnant.
   b. Her husband beat her and kicked her in the abdomen.
   c. Her children are home alone.
   d. Her mother was beaten by her father.

3. The first step in crisis intervention is assessing the patient in five important areas. Based on your review of the Nursing Admission, what assessment information did the nurse obtain in each of the following areas regarding Dorothy Grant's abuse by her husband?

Elements of Crisis Intervention Assessment	Assessment Data Found
Precipitating event	
Perception of the event by the patient	
Support system of the patient	
Coping resources of the patient	
Coping mechanisms of the patient	

4. Given Dorothy Grant's perception of the event and her coping mechanisms, what crisis intervention techniques might work best at this time?

5. Provide one example of how the nurse could help Dorothy Grant regain her self-worth.

Mental Health Promotion, Illness Prevention, Rehabilitation, and Recovery in the Hospital and Community

Reading Assignment: Mental Health Promotion and Illness Prevention (Chapter 13)
Psychiatric Rehabilitation and Recovery (Chapter 15)
Hospital-Based Psychiatric Nursing Care (Chapter 33)
Community-Based Psychiatric Nursing Care (Chapter 34)

Patient: Harry George, Medical-Surgical Floor, Room 401

Goal: To understand the role of the nurse in the continuum of care of a complex patient across treatment settings.

Objectives:

- Understand primary prevention models from different perspectives.
- Discuss the strategies used by the nurse in primary prevention.
- Describe the levels of primary prevention.
- Discuss the differences between the rehabilitation and recovery models.
- Understand the steps involved in assessing a patient's need for rehabilitation and recovery.
- Discuss the community's influence on rehabilitation and recovery.
- Understand the role of the nurse in caring for a complex patient with both chronic medical and mental health problems.
- Discuss evidenced-based community treatment interventions that help patients with substance abuse disorders.

In this lesson you will learn about the role of the nurse in the continuum of care from mental health promotion and illness prevention to hospitalization and aftercare treatment options in the community.

Exercise 1

Clinical Preparation: Writing Activity

30 minutes

1. Match each primary prevention model with its definition.

Primary Prevention Model	**Definition**
_____ Public health	a. Promotes mental health and prevention of mental illness by focusing on risk factors, vulnerability, and human response. The "patient" may be the individual, the family, or the community.
_____ Medical	
_____ Nursing	
	b. The "patient" is the community, so the emphasis is on reducing the risk for mental illness for an entire population by providing services to the high-risk group.
	c. Focuses on biological and brain research to discover specific causes of mental illness in the individual patient.

2. In planning strategies for primary prevention, the nurse uses the four interventions of

_____, _____, _____, and

_____.

3. Match each primary prevention planning strategy to its intended purpose.

Planning Strategy	**Purpose**
_____ Health education	a. Strengthens supports to increase their protective factor
_____ Environmental change	
_____ Social support	b. Dispels myths and stereotypes associated with vulnerable populations
_____ Stigma reduction	c. Helps to strengthen confidence in the patient
	d. Modification of the person's social/living situation to increase nurturing and positive reinforcement for the individual

4. Psychiatric rehabilitation is the process of helping a person return to the highest possible level of functioning. Compare and contrast psychiatric rehabilitation and recovery tertiary prevention models in terms of their definition, philosophy, and key characteristics.

Model	Definition	Philosophy	Characteristics
Psychiatric rehabilitation			
Psychiatric recovery			

Nurses need to be aware of the range of patient care needs before, during, and after hospitalization.

5. In psychiatric rehabilitation and recovery, tertiary prevention is defined as the _____

_____. The concepts of tertiary

prevention are especially relevant to those individuals with _____.

6. Name at least one agency or service in your community that provides services to the mentally ill or to those with substance abuse disorders.

Exercise 2

 CD-ROM Activity

 45 minutes

- Sign in to work at Pacific View Regional Hospital on the Medical-Surgical Floor for Period of Care 1. (*Note:* If you are already in the virtual hospital from a previous exercise, click on **Leave the Floor** and then **Restart the Program** to get to the sign-in window.)
- Select Harry George in Room 401.
- Click on **Go to Nurses' Station**.
- Click on **Chart** and then on **401**.
- Click on and read the **History and Physical**.
- Click on and read the **Nursing Assessment**.

1. Using the Nursing Prevention Model, what are the stressors that led up to Harry George's current life situation?
   a. Motorcycle accident
   b. Chronic left foot bone infection and severe pain
   c. Estrangement from his wife and two sons
   d. Loss of job
   e. Homelessness
   f. All of the above

2. What stage of prevention activities would the nurse employ during Harry George's stay in the hospital?
   a. Primary (health promotion)
   b. Secondary (crisis intervention)
   c. Tertiary (rehabilitation and recovery)

3. Match the types of health education interventions to the specific health topics Harry George will need to explore during his hospitalization and after discharge.

Type of Health Education Interventions	Specific Health Topic
_____ Increase awareness of issues related to health and illness	a. Developing healthy coping skills such as stress reduction, developing motivation and self esteem, problem-solving, and stress management
_____ Increase understanding of potential stressors, possible outcomes, and alternative coping responses	
_____ Increase knowledge of where and how to obtain resources	b. Learning how becoming clean and sober, caring for self, managing pain and diabetes, and smoking cessation can positively affect health
_____ Increase actual abilities	c. Finding housing, finding/keeping job, and locating family members
	d. Dealing with loss of family and job, homelessness, and pain

4. How important is pain management in Harry George's rehabilitation and recovery? Explain.

5. In view of Harry George's current living situation and 4-year history of alcoholism, what do you think would be the best type of program to help him quit drinking upon discharge?
   a. Community-based sober living house
   b. In-patient alcohol/drug treatment program
   c. Out-patient visits with a drug/alcohol counselor
   d. Does not really matter since he will will not stop drinking

6. What challenges does Harry George face in his recovery in the following areas of his life?

Area of Rehabilitation/Recovery	Challenge
Activities of daily living (ADL)	
Interpersonal relationships	
Self-esteem	
Motivation	
Illness management	
Strengths	

7. What available hospital-based resources can the nurse utilize to help Harry George with the community needs he will have after discharge?

8. Using information from your textbook and taking into consideration Harry George's history and current needs, discuss how a positive change in his living/social environment could affect his rehabilitation and recovery.

LESSON **7** _____

Patients with Anxiety Responses and Disorders

_____

👓 **Reading Assignment:** Anxiety Responses and Anxiety Disorders (Chapter 16)

Patient: Dorothy Grant, Obstetrics Floor, Room 201

Goal: To participate in the care of a patient on an obstetrics floor who is experiencing anxiety.

Objectives:

- Define anxiety and its essential features.
- Define types of anxiety disorders.
- Understand levels of anxiety.
- Assess physiological responses to anxiety.
- Discuss brain chemistry as it relates to anxiety.
- Understand types of events leading to anxiety.
- Discuss constructive and destructive reactions to anxiety.
- Describe outcomes associated with anxiety.
- Knowledge of medications prescribed for patients with anxiety.
- Discuss levels of anxiety as they relate to nursing interventions.
- Develop treatment interventions and outcomes for a patient with anxiety.

Exercise 1

 Clinical Preparation: Writing Activity

 30 minutes

    1. _____ is a diffuse, vague feeling of apprehension that includes feelings of uncertainty and helplessness.

2. Match each level of anxiety to its characteristics.

Level	Characteristic
_____ Mild	a. The perceptual field narrows as the person focuses on the immediate concerns
_____ Moderate	b. Associated with dread and terror; the personality becomes disorganized
_____ Severe	c. Associated with the tension of daily life
_____ Panic	d. Significant reduction in the perceptual field as the person focuses on details and cannot think of anything else

3. Identify at least two physiological responses to anxiety in each of the systems below.

System	Physiological Responses
Cardiovascular	
Respiratory	
Gastrointestinal	
Neuromuscular	
Urinary tract	
Skin	

4. Match each type of response to anxiety with its group of characteristics.

Type of Response	**Characteristics**
_____ Behavioral	a. Loss of objectiveness, poor concentration, preoccupation, thought blocking, decreased productivity
_____ Cognitive	
_____ Affective	b. Uneasiness, nervousness, impatience, jumpiness, fear, fright
	c. Rapid speech, restlessness, tremors, physical tension, hyperventilation

5. The biological basis of anxiety involves three neurotransmitters in the brain. Explain the role each neurotransmitter plays in anxiety.

Neurotransmitter	**Role in Anxiety**
GABA	
Norepinephrine	
Serotonin	

6. _____ reactions to anxiety are thoughtful, deliberate attempts to solve

   problems, resolve conflicts, and gratify needs, whereas _____ reactions, also

   called _____ are often used to protect a person and are the
   first line of defense to successfully cope with mild to moderate anxiety.

7. Discuss three important nursing interventions in working with a patient with severe and
   panic levels of anxiety.

Exercise 2

 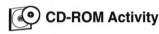 **CD-ROM Activity**

30 minutes

- Sign in to work at Pacific View Regional Hospital on the Obstetrics Floor for Period of Care 1. (*Note:* If you are already in the virtual hospital from a previous exercise, click on **Leave the Floor** and then **Restart the Program** to get to the sign-in window.)
- Select Dorothy Grant in Room 201
- Click on **Get Report**.

1. According to the change-of-shift report, what level of anxiety is Dorothy Grant experiencing?
   a. Mild
   b. Moderate
   c. Severe
   d. Panic

2. It is reported that Dorothy Grant's stated concerns of _____ and the

   _____ are causing her anxiety.

 • Now click on **Return to Patient List** and then on **Go to Nurses' Station**.
- Click on Room **201** at the bottom of the screen.
- Click on **Patient Care**.
- Click on **Nurse-Client Interactions**.
- Select and view the video titled **0730: Patient Teaching—Medication**. (*Note:* If this video is not available, check the virtual clock to see whether enough time has elapsed. The video cannot be viewed before its specified time.)

3. How does the nurse's assessment of Dorothy Grant's anxiety level compare with assessment described in the change-of-shift report?

 • Now click on **Chart** and then on **201**.
- Access and read the **Nursing Assessment** section.

4. What are the two stressors listed that contribute to Dorothy Grant's anxiety?

5. Precipitating stressors can be grouped into two categories: threats to physical integrity and threats to self-system. How would you describe Dorothy Grant's stressors in terms of these two categories?

6. Dorothy Grant has been using maladaptive or destructive coping mechanisms to handle her stressors. Next to each destructive or maladaptive coping mechanism listed below, identify an alternative constructive or adaptive mechanism.

Maladaptive (Destructive) Coping Mechanism	Adaptive (Constructive) Coping Mechanism
Hoping the abuse will stop	
Keeping the children quiet	
Blaming herself for causing the abuse (pregnancy)	
Trying not to upset husband	

7. You have assessed Dorothy Grant's level of anxiety to be moderate in severity. Develop nursing interventions based on the following aspects of treatment.

Aspects	Nursing Interventions
Recognition	
Insight	
Education	
Coping	

→ • Click on **Return to Room 201**.
• Now click on **MAR** and review Dorothy Grant's medications.
• Check to see whether there are any medications ordered for Dorothy Grant's anxiety.

8. What classification of medications would be ordered for a patient with moderate to severe anxiety?
a. Antidepressants
b. Antianxiety agents
c. Antipsychotics
d. Stimulants

9. In deciding whether to order medication to treat Dorothy Grant's anxiety, what are the key considerations?
a. 30 weeks pregnant/possible contraindications
b. Anxiety initially assessed to be at a moderate level
c. Blunt force trauma to abdomen/may result in preterm delivery
d. Need more time to assess patient's anxiety
e. All of the above

10. The best treatment outcomes will demonstrate adaptive ways of coping with stress. From the list below, choose two treatment outcome statements that best describe desired outcomes based on Dorothy Grant's treatment plan. (*Hint:* See Box 16-8, Outcome Indicators for Anxiety Self-Control, in your textbook.)

_____ a. Maintains adequate sleep

_____ b. Plans coping strategies for stressful situations

_____ c. Monitors behavioral manisfestations of anxiety

_____ d. Eliminates precursors of anxiety

Patients with Emotional Responses and Mood Disorders

Reading Assignment: Self-Protective Responses and Suicidal Behavior (Chapter 19)

Patient: Kelly Brady, Obstetrics Floor, Room 203

Goal: To care for a patient who is experiencing a medical health crisis (severe preeclampsia at 26 weeks gestation) and also has symptoms of depression.

Objectives:

- Understand depression in the context of the continuum of emotional responses.
- Assess a patient who is demonstrating an unhealthy emotional state.
- Identify behaviors associated with depression.
- Discuss the risk for suicide in patients with severe mood disturbance.
- Understand the relationship between depressed mood and pregnancy.
- Describe predisposing risk factors and precipitaing stressors in depression.
- Identify coping resources and mechanisms of patients with depression.
- Describe effective interventions including pharmacological treatment for depressed patients.
- Develop a treatment plan for a patient with depression.

Exercise 1

 Clinical Preparation: Writing Activity

🕐 30 minutes

1. Using the continuum of emotional responses in your textbook, match the specific response on the left to the type of response on the right.

Response	**Type of Response**
_____ Emotional responsiveness	a. Adaptive or maladaptive
_____ Uncomplicated grief reaction	b. Maladaptive
_____ Suppression of emotions	c. Adaptive
_____ Delayed grief reaction	
_____ Depression or mania	

2. Select the correct fact(s) about depression.
   a. 1 in 5 patients seen by their primary provider have significant symptoms of depression.
   b. Major depression accounts for more days spent home in bed than any other physical illness except cardiovascular disease.
   c. Major depression is more costly to our economy than chronic respiratory disease, diabetes, arthritis, or hypertension.
   d. 85% of patients with depression can be treated successfully using a combination of verbal therapies and medication.
   e. All of the above

3. Complete the table below by listing examples of symptoms associated with persons with depression.

Symptoms	Examples
Affective	
Physiological	
Cognitive	
Behavioral	

4. Genetics plays an important role in depression. What is the lifetime risk for relatives of people with depression to experience depression themselves?
   a. 5%
   b. 10%
   c. 20%
   d. 30%

5. People with depression have a genuine need to believe that things can get better. To help patients with this need, the nurse:
   a. must initially express hope to the patient.
   b. reinforce the fact that depression is a self-limiting disorder and the future will be better.
   c. explain to the patient that depression is a chronic disease.
   d. should do a and b only.

6. There is evidence that shows cognitive therapy to be an effective treatment for depression.

   The three objectives of cognitive behavioral strategies are _____

   _____, _____, and _____

   _____.

7. Successful behavior is a powerful tool to counteract depression. Discuss specific interventions the nurse can implement in caring for the depressed patient to effect positive behavioral change. Include three activities that the patient can accomplish to make positive behavioral changes.

8. For treating patients with depression, which class of medications has proven the most effective with the least amount of side effects?
   a. Selective serotonin reuptake inhibitors (SSRIs)
   b. Monoamine oxidase inhibitors (MAOIs)
   c. Tricyclic antidepressant drugs (TCAs)

9. How would the nurse educate the depressed patient on the importance of developing increased social skills?

10. List the four underlying principles that govern a psychoeducational program on depression for patients and their families.

Exercise 2

 CD-ROM Activity

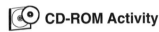 30 minutes

- Sign in to work at Pacific View Regional Hospital on the Obstetrics Floor for Period of Care 1. (*Note:* If you are already in the virtual hospital from a previous exercise, click on **Leave the Floor** and then **Restart the Program** to get to the sign-in window.)
- Select Kelly Brady in Room 203.
- Click on **Get Report**. After reading report, click on **Return to Patient List**.
- Click on **Go to Nurses' Station**.
- Click on **203** at the bottom of the screen.
- Inside the patient's room, click on **Patient Care** and then on **Physical Assessment**.
- Click on **Head & Neck**.
- Click on **Mental Status**.

1. Based on the mental status assessment, Kelly Brady's two documented behavioral symp-

   toms are _____ and _____.

- Now click on **Chart** and then on **203**.
- Click on and read the **History and Physical**.

2. The predisposing factor in Kelly Brady's family history related to depression is

   _____. In her past medical history, the key

   fact related to depression is _____.

3. Kelly Brady had a diagnosed episode of depression in college. What percentage of those who have had depression in the past will eventually have it again?
   a. 10%
   b. 25%
   c. 50%
   d. 75%

- Still in the chart, click on **Mental Health** and read the Psychiatric Mental Health Assessment.
- Then click on **Consultations** and read the Psychiatric Consult.

4. According to the DSM IV Axis I diagnosis and her symptoms, where on the emotional response continuum does Kelly Brady fall?
   a. Emotional responsiveness
   b. Uncomplicated grief reaction
   c. Suppression of emotions
   d. Delayed grief reaction
   e. Depression

5. The continuum of emotional responses range from adaptive to maladaptive. The type of

   emotional response Kelly Brady is using is _____.

6. What major life events/precipitating stressors are contributing to Kelly Brady's mood disturbance?
   a. Lack of supports: mother has cancer, parents out of town, and sister going through divorce
   b. Financial stress: problems with her and husband's job and moving into larger home
   c. Biological factors: pregnancy
   d. All of the above

7. List all the behavioral symptoms Kelly Brady is experiencing related to depression.

8. To begin developing a treatment plan to address Kelly Brady's depression, complete the intervention section of the treatment plan below.

Area	Goal	Intervention
Environment/safety	To keep patient safe	
Cognitive	To move patient beyond her preoccupation to other aspects of her life	
Behavioral	To accomplish tasks and activities to counteract depression	
Social skills	To provide experiences to counteract depression and social isolation and build self-esteem	
Education	To educate the patient about depression and the interventions and treatment that will be helpful	

9. Discuss how Kelly Brady's pregnancy might be related to her depression.

10. Kelly Brady's physician has recommended that she take paroxetine after the birth of her baby. From the records you have read, fill in the blanks below.

The trade name for paroxetine is _____, and the dose that was recom-

mended was _____. The clinical rationale for recommending paroxetine is that

_____.

Patients with Neurobiological Responses and Thought Disorders

 Reading Assignment: Neurobiological Responses and Schizophrenia and
Psychotic Disorders (Chapter 20)

Patient: Jacquline Catanazaro, Medical-Surgical Floor, Room 402

Goal: To care for a patient with chronic schizophrenia who is hospitalized for acute asthma.

Objectives:

- Understand the range of neurobiological responses from adaptive to maladaptive and know where schizophrenia is located within the range.
- Understand the meaning of psychosis and its symptomatology.
- List the positive and negative symptoms of schizophrenia.
- Understand symptoms of schizophrenia in terms of their impact on the cognitive, perceptual, emotional, behavioral, and social aspects of the person's life.
- Identify predisposing factors and precipitating stressors of schizophrenia and understand how to appraise stressors.
- Identify coping resources the person with schizophrenia has available and recognize the coping mechanisms they are utilizing.
- Understand the components of an education plan for a patient with schizophrenia.
- Identify the components of discharge planning for a patient with schizophrenia.

Exercise 1

 Clinical Preparation: Writing Activity

15 minutes

1. _____ refers to the mental state of experiencing reality differently from others;

   _____ is a serious and persistent neurobiological brain disease that includes profoundly disruptive psychopathology that severely impairs the lives of individuals, their families, and communities.

2. In the continuum of neurobiological responses, schizophrenia would be considered a

_____ response.

3. The impact of schizophrenia on the individual and society is enormous. Place an X next to the true statements about schizophrenia.

_____ a. In the United States, about 2.5 million people suffer from schizophrenia (roughly 1 of every 100 Americans).

_____ b. Of people diagnosed with schizophrenia, 100% have the disease for life.

_____ c. In 75% of cases, the onset for schizophrenia is between the ages of 17 and 25.

_____ d. 33% to 50% of homeless people in the United States have schizophrenia.

_____ e. Schizophrenia ranks tenth in the world in terms of burden of illness.

_____ f. 20% to 50% of patients with schizophrenia attempt suicide, and between 9% and 13% succeed.

4. It is important to understand and differentiate the positive and negative symptoms of schizophrenia. Identify the positive and negative symptoms associated with the categories listed below.

Categories	Positive Symptoms	Negative Symptoms
Thinking		
Emotion		
Speech		
Behavior		
Response to medication		

5. Numerous stressors or triggers often precede a new episode or exacerbation of the symptoms of schizophrenia. Match each of the following triggers to its corresponding category.

Common Relapse Trigger	Category of Stressor
_____ Low self-concept/self-confidence	a. Health
_____ Lack of social support	b. Environment
_____ Housing difficulties	c. Attitudes
_____ Aggressive/violent behavior	d. Behavior
_____ Lack of sleep	
_____ Poor medication management	
_____ Lack of transportation	
_____ Financial problems	
_____ Job pressures	
_____ Poor nutrition	
_____ Social isolation	
_____ Interpersonal difficulties	

Exercise 2

 CD-ROM Activity

 45 minutes

- Sign in to work at Pacific View Regional Hospital on the Medical-Surgical Floor for Period of Care 3. (*Note:* If you are already in the virtual hospital from a previous exercise, click on **Leave the Floor** and then **Restart the Program** to get to the sign-in window.)
- Select Jacquline Catanazaro in Room 402.
- Click on **Go to Nurses' Station**.
- Click on **Chart** and then on **402**.
- Click on **Nurse's Notes**.
- Read the note written on admission on Monday at 1600.

1. Identify two pieces of information contained in the nurse's admission note that have implications for discharge planning.
    a. Patient has asthma.
    b. Sister is patient's main support.
    c. Patient has no transportation.
    d. Patient has a history of stopping her psychiatric medication.
    e. b and d only

➜ • Now read the **Nurse's Notes** dated Tuesday at 0400.

2. The statement made by the patient that people are putting poison into her IV is an example of what type of delusion?
   a. Grandiose
   b. Persecutory
   c. Paranoid
   d. None of the above

➜ • Now read the **Nurse's Notes** dated Wednesday at 0600.

3. The note describes symptoms of schizophrenia that have a direct relationship to Jacquline Catanazaro's asthma. Explain the relationship.

➜ • Now click on the **Consultation** tab in the chart.
   • Read the Psychiatric Consult.

4. The positive symptom of schizophrenia described in the report is _____,

   and the negative symptoms described are _____ and _____

   _____.

5. The plan contained within the Psychiatric Consult includes exercise and nutrition. Comment on the relevance of diet and exercise as part of the plan of care for Jacquline Catanazaro.

➜ • Click on and review the **History and Physical** and **Nursing Admission** sections.

6. For each category below, list Jacquline Catanazaro's barriers to compliance that may result in future relapses.

Category	Barriers to Compliance
Health	
Thoughts	
Attitudes	
Behavior	
Socialization	
Medication	

7. Education will be a critical component of Jacquline Catanazaro's treatment plan. Place an X next to each of her educational needs.

_____ a. Healthy living

_____ b. Medication

_____ c. Psychoeducation

_____ d. Illness management

→ • Click on **Return to Nurses' Station**.
 • Click on **MAR** and then on tab **402**.
 • Scroll down to locate the antipsychotic medication ordered.
 • Click on **Return to Nurses' Station**.
 • Click on the **Drug** icon in the lower left corner of the screen. Find the entry for this medication.

8. Based on your review of the Drug Guide, fill in the information requested below.

Name of medication

Indication

Mechanism of action

Side effects

Dosage

Nursing considerations

Patient teaching

9. Review the medication dosage Jacquline Catanazaro is receiving and the usual dosage as stated in the Drug Guide. What might be the rationale for the current dosage the physician is giving to her?

• Click on **Return to Nurses' Station**.
 • Click on the **402** to go to the patient's room.
 • Click on **Patient Care**.
 • Click on **Nurse-Client Interactions**.
 • Select and view the video titled **1500: Intervention—Patient Teaching**.
 • After watching the 1500 video, select and view the video titled **1540: Discharge Planning**. (*Note:* If this video is not available, check the virtual clock to see whether enough time has elapsed. The video cannot be viewed before its specified time.)

10. Discuss the importance of including Jacquline Catanazaro's sister in the discharge planning process.

Patients with Cognitive Responses, Organic Mental Disorders, and Aggressive Behavior

Reading Assignment: Cognitive Responses and Organic Mental Disorders (Chapter 22)

Preventing and Managing Aggressive Behavior (Chapter 29)

Patient: Carlos Reyes, Skilled Nursing Floor, Room 504

Goal: To care for a patient who has symptoms of cardiovascular disease and cognitive impairment, including agitation.

Objectives:

- Recognize the continuum of adaptive and maladaptive cognitive responses.
- Compare and contrast definitions and characteristics of delirium and dementia.
- Provide examples of severe disturbed behavior associated with dementia.
- Identify structures in the brain responsible for aggressive behavior that often accompany maladaptive cognitive responses.
- Identify precipitating stressors associated with delirium and dementia.
- Discuss the high-priority nursing interventions in working with patients with delirium and dementia.
- Describe medications used in the treatment of dementia and agitation.
- Identify underlying medical conditions that can produce symptoms of delirium.
- Understand family involvement in discharge planning, including cultural aspects of care.

Exercise 1

Clinical Preparation: Writing Activity

15 minutes

1. Maladaptive cognitive responses include which of the following? Place an X next to all that apply.

_____ a. Inability to make decisions

_____ b. Impaired memory and judgment

_____ c. Oriented to person, time, and place

_____ d. Misperceptions

_____ e. Attention to detail

_____ f. Difficulty with logical reasoning

2. Maladaptive cognitive responses are most apparent in people who have a diagnosis of
   a. delirium.
   b. dementia.
   c. a and b.

3. Delirium is characterized by the _____ of awareness and a _____

   onset, whereas dementia is characterized by the loss of _____ abilities of

   _____, _____, and _____, and has a

   _____ onset.

4. In addition to the usual dementia symptoms of disorientation, confusion, memory loss, disorganized thinking, and poor judgment, some patients may experience more severe disturbed behavior. Match the following categories and examples of behavior.

Category of Behavior	**Example of Behavior**
_____ Aggressive psychomotor behavior	a. Incontinence, poor hygiene
_____ Nonaggressive psychomotor behavior	b. Demanding, complaining, screaming, disruptive
_____ Verbally aggressive behavior	c. Decreased activity, apathy, withdrawal
_____ Passive behavior	d. Hitting, kicking, pushing, scratching, assaultive
_____ Functionally impaired behavior	e. Restless, pacing, wandering

5. There are three structures in the brain implicated in aggressive behavior: the frontal lobe, limbic system, and hypothalamus. List the function and dysfunction of each area below.

Area of Brain	Function	Dysfunction
Frontal lobe		
Limbic system		
Hypothalamus		

6. Any major disregulation in the balance of body functions can disrupt cognitive functioning. Discuss cardiac disorders and cardiac medications as potential precipitating stressors in delirium.

7. In caring for the patient experiencing symptoms of delerium, the highest priority is given to

nursing interventions that _____. Three nursing interventions that maintain life

are _____, _____

_____, and _____

_____.

8. In providing care to patients with dementia, the highest priority is given to nursing interventions that maintain the patient's optimum level of functioning. Complete the table below

Component of Care	Interventions
Social interaction	
Medications	
Orientation	
Communication	
Wandering	
Agitation	
Family and community	

Exercise 2

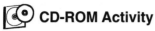 **CD-ROM Activity**

 30 minutes

- Sign in to work at Pacific View Regional Hospital on the Skilled Nursing Floor Floor for Period of Care 2. (*Note:* If you are already in the virtual hospital from a previous exercise, click on **Leave the Floor** and then **Restart the Program** to get to the sign-in window.)
- Select Carlos Reyes in Room 504.
- Click on **Get Report**.
- Read both shift summaries on the Clinical Report.

  1. According to the shift reports, Carlos Reyes' most problematic symptoms have been

     _____, _____,

     and _____.

- Now click on **Return to Patient List** and then **Go to Nurses' Station**.
- Click on Room **504** at the bottom of the screen.
- Click on **Patient Care**.
- Click on **Physical Assessment**.
- Click on **Head & Neck**.
- Click on and read **Mental Status**.

  2. During the mental status assessment, what symptoms are described that indicate Carlos Reyes is having maladaptive cognitive responses?

  3. In the list below, place an X next to the behaviors Carlos Reyes is exhibiting that are associated with aggression.

     _____ a. Extreme anxiety

     _____ b. Irritability

     _____ c. Soft-spoken

     _____ d. Confusion

     _____ e. Memory intact

     _____ f. Disorientation

• Now click on **Nurse-Client Interactions**.
 • Select and view the video titled **1120: The Agitated Patient**. (*Note:* If this video is not available, check the virtual clock to see whether enough time has elapsed. The video cannot be viewed before its specified time.)

4. Select the intervention(s) the nurse used to respond to Carlos Reyes' agitation.
 a. Ignored the difficult behavior
 b. Listened to the patient and patient's daughter
 c. Spoke in a calm, reassuring manner to decrease stress in the environment
 d. Modified the original plan to meet the patient's needs
 e. Did all except a

 • Now select and view the video titled **1140: Assessing for Referrals**.

5. Assess the son's understanding of Carlos Reyes' illness. What action will the nurse need to take after her brief interaction with his son?

Exercise 3

 CD-ROM Activity

 30 minutes

 • Sign in to work at Pacific View Regional Hospital on the Skilled Nursing Floor for Period of Care 3. (*Note:* If you are already in the virtual hospital from a previous exercise, click on **Leave the Floor** and then **Restart the Program** to get to the sign-in window.)
 • Select Carlos Reyes in Room 504.
 • Click on **Go to Nurses' Station**.
 • Click on **Chart** and then on **504**.
 • Read the **History and Physical**.
 • Read the **Nursing Admission**.

1. If Carlos Reyes returns to his daughter's home after discharge, discuss the problems that his daughter may have in caring for him.

2. Now that you have reviewed all the pertinent data, what factors may be contributing to Carlos Reyes' confusion? Place an X next to all that apply.

_____ a. Change in environment

_____ b. Recent MI

_____ c. History of dementia

_____ d. Medication regime

→ • Click on **Return to Nurses' Station**.
 • Click on **504** to go to Carlos Reyes' room.
 • Inside the room, click on **Patient Care** and then on **Nurse-Client Interactions**.
 • Select and view the video titled **1500: The Confused Patient**.

3. Describe the approach the nurse used in dealing with Carlos Reyes' confusion.

→ • Now select and view the video titled **1505: Family Teaching—Dementia**.

4. In the interaction with Carlos Reyes' daughter, describe the intervention the nurse used.

→ • Click on **MAR** and select tab **504**.
 • Review the medication ordered for anxiety and agitation.
 • Click on **Return to Room 504**.
 • Click on the **Drug** icon in the lower left corner of the screen.
 • Find and review this medication in the Drug Guide.

5. To identify the important aspects of this medication, provide the information requested below and on the next page.

Name of medication

Class

Mechanism of action

Therapeutic effect

Indication

Dosage

Side effects

Nursing indications

 • Again click on **Return to Room 504**.
   • Click on **Patient Care**.
   • Click on **Nurse-Client Interactions**.
   • Select and view the video titled **1525: Family Conflict—Discharge Plan**. (*Note:* If this
      video is not available, check the virtual clock to see whether enough time has elapsed. The
      video cannot be viewed before its specified time.)
   • After observing the interaction, click on **Chart** and then on **504**.
   • Click on **Consultations**.
   • Read the Discharge Coordinator Consult.

   6. Describe the family conflict associated with Carlos Reyes' care, its implication with regard
      to discharge planning, and how the nurse should best approach the situation.

7. In successful discharge planning, practical recommendations are necessary for caregivers who must care for family members with dementia, especially those who are also agitated and aggressive. Using your textbook and what you know about Carlos Reyes, provide some practical approaches below that you believe would be helpful to his daughter.

Area of Focus	Practical Approaches
Decrease escalation	
Communicate effectively	
Review the basics	

Patients with Chemically Mediated Responses and Substance-Related Disorders

/oo **Reading Assignment:** Chemically Mediated Responses and Substance-Related Disorders (Chapter 23)

Patient: Laura Wilson, Obstetrics Floor, Room 206

Goal: To care for a patient with acute medical needs who also has a diagnosis of polysubstance abuse.

Objectives:

- Describe the continuum of adaptive and maladaptive chemically mediated responses.
- Understand behaviors of abuse and dependence.
- Describe predisposing factors, precipitating stressors, and appraisal of stressors related to substance abuse.
- Examine the nurse's own feelings about working with a patient who is pregnant and HIV-positive and has polysubstance abuse.
- Identify nursing diagnosis as it relates to polysubstance abuse.
- Identify key aspects of the treatment plan to include patient teaching for a patient with poly-substance abuse.
- Discuss issues involved in discharge planning of a patient who has polysubstance abuse.

Exercise 1

 Clinical Preparation: Writing Activity

 15 minutes

1. Drugs that affect the pleasure centers of the _____ and therefore create

   pleasurable changes in the mental and emotional states have the greatest potential for

   _____. _____ is a very popular drug of abuse because it produces
   effects on the brain within minutes.

103

2. Identify the potential drugs of abuse in the following list. Place an X next to all that apply.

   _____ a. Alcohol

   _____ b. Cocaine

   _____ c. Marijuana

   _____ d. Prescription pain medications

   _____ e. Heroin

   _____ f. Inhalants

   _____ g. Prescription diet pills

   _____ h. Prescription antianxiety medications

3. Not everyone who uses drugs becomes an abuser; however, for some users, the range of

   chemically mediated coping responses begins with _____

   and progresses to _____ and eventually leads to

   _____ and _____.

4. Terms of abuse are important to understand when discussing chemically mediated coping responses. Match each term with its corresponding definition.

Terms	**Definition**
_____ Substance abuse	a. The psychosocial behaviors related to substance dependence
_____ Substance dependence	b. Occurs when there is a coexistence of substance abuse and a psychiatric disorder
_____ Addiction	
_____ Dual diagnosis	c. Includes withdrawal symptoms and tolerance of substance
_____ Physical dependence	d. Continued use of substances despite related problems
_____ Withdrawal symptoms	
_____ Tolerance	e. Severe condition usually considered a disease that may include physical problems and serious disruption in the person's life
	f. Result from a biological need that occurs when the body becomes used to having the substance in the system
	g. Occurs with continued use, as more of the substance is needed to produce the same effect

5. Discuss the importance of drug testing of patients who present with substance abuse.

6. Lifestyles associated with substance abuse carry risks. Select the lifestyle risks associated with substance abuse.
   a. Accidents
   b. Violence
   c. Self-neglect
   d. Physical and mental illnesses
   e. Complications during pregnancy
   f. Fetal abnormalities and substance dependence
   g. Hepatitis B and C
   h. HIV and AIDS
   i. All of the above

7. In terms of the predisposing factors of substance abuse, several models have been proposed within the biological, psychological, and sociocultural spheres. Since a belief in a particular model influences the way in which the nurse thinks about and will work with the patient, discuss your beliefs about persons with substance abuse.

Exercise 2

 CD-ROM Activity

 15 minutes

- Sign in to work at Pacific View Regional Hospital on the Obstetrics Floor for Period of Care 1. (*Note:* If you are already in the virtual hospital from a previous exercise, click on **Leave the Floor** and then **Restart the Program** to get to the sign-in window.)
- Select Laura Wilson in Room 206
- Click on **Get Report**.
- After reading the report, click on **Return to Patient List** and then click on **Go to Nurses' Station**.
- Click on **Chart** and then on **206**.
- Click on **Emergency Department** and read the report.

1. What information lets the nurse know that Laura Wilson may be abusing drugs?
   a. Found unconscious
   b. Nausea and diarrhea
   c. HIV-positive status
   d. History of drug abuse
   e. a and d only

2. Laura Wilson's urine drug screen came back positive for THC and cocaine. Complete the table below regarding the characteristics of these two drugs.

Substance	Route	Signs and Symptoms of Use	Withdrawal Signs and Symptoms	Consequences of Use
Cocaine				
Marijuana				

→ • Click on **Nursing Admission** tab.
  • Read the report.

3. In addition to caffeine, there are two other drugs Laura Wilson is abusing. The report indi-

   cates they are _____ and _____.

4. Explain how these drugs might affect the health of her baby.

5. The Nursing Admission record contains information regarding Laura Wilson's precipitating stressors. Place an X next to the stressors Laura Wilson has identified.

   _____ a. Parents disapproval of her lifestyle

   _____ b. HIV-positive status

   _____ c. Unplanned pregnancy

   _____ d. Desire to quit "crack"

   _____ e. Boyfriend out of town

6. Select the best coping resource that might be available to Laura Wilson.
   a. Younger sister
   b. Boyfriend
   c. Mother and father
   d. Roommate

7. Laura Wilson's most frequently used coping mechanisms for dealing with her problems are

   _____ and _____.

Exercise 3

 CD-ROM Activity

 30 minutes

• Sign in to work at Pacific View Regional Hospital on the Obstetrics Floor for Period of Care 2. (*Note:* If you are already in the virtual hospital from a previous exercise, click on **Leave the Floor** and then **Restart the Program** to get to the sign-in window.)
• Select Laura Wilson in Room 206.
• Click on **Get Report**.
• Click on **Return to Patient List** and then on **Go to Nurses' Station**.
• Click on Room **206** at the bottom of the screen.
• Click on **Patient Care**.
• Click on **Nurse-Client Interactions**.
• Select and view the video titled **1115: Teaching—Effects of Drug Use**. (*Note:* If this video is not available, check the virtual clock to see whether enough time has elapsed. The video cannot be viewed before its specified time.)

1. Which statements made by Laura Wilson during the interaction best illustrate her lack of understanding regarding substance abuse?
   a. "The baby will help me stay on track."
   b. "It's not like I'm addicted. I can quit anytime."
   c. "It's not like the baby will be addicted."
   d. "I have to quit for a month or two."
   e. All except d

2. Place an X next to the statement(s) that may indicate Laura Wilson's readiness to abstain from drugs.

   _____ a. "It wasn't a hard decision for me. I am looking forward to this baby."

   _____ b. "I can go for a while without taking drugs."

   _____ c. "My mom doesn't believe I can do it."

   _____ d. "I'll do whatever it takes to keep my baby."

3. What do you see as the barriers to Laura Wilson's abstinence from drugs?

4. Evaluate the nurse's role in educating Laura Wilson on the effects of drug use.

→ • Click on **MAR**.
   • Find the medication ordered for Laura Wilson's pain.
   • Click on the **Drug** icon in the lower left corner of the screen.
   • Locate and review the entry for this medication.

5. The medication ordered for Laura Wilson's pain is _____. In her situation,

   the two most important features of this medication are _____

   and _____.

6. An important aspect of Laura Wilson's treatment plan will be the teaching plan. Match her education needs and the interventions that will best help her.

Education Needs	**Effective Interventions**
_____ HIV-positive	a. Well-baby clinic and parental support
_____ Caring for her newborn	b. Community AA-based self-help group and individual motivational and cognitive behavioral approaches
_____ Drug abstinence	
_____ Handling family conflict	c. HIV counselor/HIV clinic
_____ Community resources	d. Consultation with hospital social worker/ discharge planner
	e. Family counseling

 7. For patients who abuse substances, a key aspect of discharge planning is a relapse prevention plan, developed together by the nurse and patient. Discuss the key elements to the relapse prevention plan for Laura Wilson. (*Hint:* See pages 504-505 in your textbook.)

LESSON 12

Patients with Eating Regulation Response and Eating Disorders

Reading Assignment: Regulation Response and Eating Disorders (Chapter 24)

Patient: Tiffany Sheldon, Pediatrics Floor, Room 305

Goal: To provide nursing care for a patient with an eating disorder who also has comorbid psychiatric symptoms.

Objectives:

* Identify behaviors associated with eating disorders.
* Describe the continuum of adaptive and maladaptive eating disorder regulation responses.
* Discuss predisposing factors and precipitating stressors related to eating disorders.
* Assess interactions between nurses and a patient with an eating disorder.
* Identify coping resources and coping mechanisms related to eating disorders.
* Assess and plan care for a patient with an eating disorder.
* Identify the psychological components of a treatment plan for a patient with an eating disorder.
* Identify outcomes for a patient with an eating disorder.

Exercise 1

Clinical Preparation: Writing Activity

15 minutes

1. Food is essential to life but can also be used to satisfy _____,

   to moderate _____, and to provide _____ and _____.

2. Place an X next to the symptoms and/or behaviors that best reflect maladaptive eating regulation response.

    _____ a. Night eating syndrome

    _____ b. Skipping meals occasionally

    _____ c. Anorexia

    _____ d. Severe dieting

    _____ e. Overeating under stress

    _____ f. Bulimia

    _____ g. Frequent fasting

    _____ h. Binge eating disorder

3. The psychological reasons for disordered eating can lead to serious biological changes such

    as _____, _____, and _____.

    Psychological problems associated with eating disorders include _____,

    _____, and _____.

4. How do sociocultural factors regarding body size affect the prevalence of eating disorders?

5. There are many factors that predispose a person to develop an eating disorder. Place an X next to the psychological symptoms associated with eating disorders.

    _____ a. Rigid, meticulous, and ritualistic behavior

    _____ b. No early childhood issues

    _____ c. Persuasive sense of ineffectiveness and helplessness

    _____ d. Understands feeling of others

    _____ e. Difficulty tolerating intense emotional states

    _____ f. Fear of biological or psychological maturity

6. Many people who are in treatment for eating disorders have evidence of other psychiatric disorders. For each type of eating disorder listed below, identify the psychiatric comorbidity.

Eating Disorder	Psychiatric Comorbidity
Anorexia	
Bulimia	
Anorexia and bulimia	
Binge eating disorder	
Night eating disorder	

7. Discuss the environmental factors that may predispose someone to an eating disorder.

8. What feelings do you have regarding those who have eating disorders that result in being severely underweight or overweight? How might sociocultural factors play a part in these feelings? Do you recognize any bias toward patients with these problems? Explain.

Exercise 2

 CD-ROM Activity

15 minutes

- Sign in to work at Pacific View Regional Hospital on the Pediatrics Floor for Period of Care 1. (*Note:* If you are already in the virtual hospital from a previous exercise, click on **Leave the Floor** and then **Restart the Program** to get to the sign-in window.)
- Select Tiffany Sheldon in Room 305.
- Click on **Get Report**.

1. Based on the shift report, the possible psychiatric behaviors Tiffany Sheldon is exhibiting

   are _____, _____, and _____.

- Click on **Return to Patient List** and then on **Go to Nurses' Station**.
- Click on Room **305** at the bottom of the screen.
- Click on **Patient Care** and then on **Physical Assessment**.
- Click on **Head & Neck**.
- Click on **Mental Status**.

2. Place an X next to the characteristics that apply to Tiffany Sheldon based on the shift report and the findings of the mental status assessment.

   _____ a. Good eye contact

   _____ b. Listless

   _____ c. Flat affect

   _____ d. Energetic

   _____ e. Avoids eye contact

   _____ f. Withdrawn

- Click on **Nurse-Client Interactions**.
- Select and view the video titled **0730: Initial Assessment**. (*Note:* If this video is not available, check the virtual clock to see whether enough time has elapsed. The video cannot be viewed before its specified time.)

3. Describe your reaction to Tiffany Sheldon's responses to the nurse who is caring for her.

→ • Click on **Chart**.
  • Click on **Physician's Orders**.

4. Which orders indicate that multidimensional assessments (in addition to physical assessments) are being implemented for Tiffany Sheldon's care?
   a. Nursing supervision during and after meals
   b. Nutritionist to follow patient
   c. Involvement of adolescent care team
   d. Involvement of eating disorders clinic
   e. Consultation with psychiatric team
   f. All of the above

→ • Click on the **History and Physical** and review.

5. Tiffany Sheldon's medical diagnoses are _____, _____, and

   _____.

→ • Click on **Nursing Admission** and review.

6. List at least two possible psychological and two environmental predisposing factors associated with Tiffany Sheldon's eating disorder.

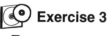 **Exercise 3**

 CD-ROM Activity

30 minutes

• Sign in to work at Pacific View Regional Hospital on the Pediatrics Floor for Period of Care 3. (*Note:* If you are already in the virtual hospital from a previous exercise, click on **Leave the Floor** and then **Restart the Program** to get to the sign-in window.)
• Select Tiffany Sheldon in Room 305.
• Click on **Get Report**.
• Click on **Return to Patient List** and then on **Go to Nurses' Station**.
• Click on Room **305** at the bottom of the screen.
• Click on **Patient Care**.
• Click on **Nurse-Client Interactions**.
• Select and view the video titled **1500: Relapse—Contributing Factors**. (*Note:* If this video is not available, check the virtual clock to see whether enough time has elapsed. The video cannot be viewed before its specified time.)

1. Tiffany Sheldon's predisposing factors make her especially vulnerable to environmental pressures and stress. Choose the stressors that have contributed to her current relapse of her eating disorder.
   a. Parents divorced 3 years ago.
   b. Family does not understand her problem.
   c. Mom is angry and "disgusted."
   d. She visited her father in Florida 2 weeks ago.
   e. c and d only

➡ • Click on **Chart** and then on **305**.
• Click on **Mental Health**.
• Read the Psychiatric Assessment.

2. Characteristic of those who have anorexia, Tiffany Sheldon's main maladaptive coping

   mechanism is _____.

3. For people with anorexia, the issue is not really about their weight, but rather about control-

   ling life and fears. Tiffany Sheldon's statement, "_____,"
   is an example of this overriding concern.

4. In addition to Tiffany Sheldon's diagnosis of imbalanced nutrition less than body require-ments, identify two nursing diagnoses that best describe the psychological components to her eating disorder.

➡ • Click on **Return to Room 305**.
• Click on **Patient Care**.
• Click on **Nurse-Client Interactions**.
• Select and view the video titled **1530: Facilitating Success**. (*Note:* If this video is not avail-able, check the virtual clock to see whether enough time has elapsed. The video cannot be viewed before its specified time.)

5. One of the most important parts in assessing a patient with an eating disorder is the person's motivation to change the behavior. What statement does Tiffany Sheldon make that best defines her motivation level and has implications for her success in preventing relapse?

➡ • Click on **Chart** and then on **305**.
• Click on **Consultations**.
• Read the Psychiatric Consult.

6. Two plans of care are being implemented simultaneously for Tiffany Sheldon. One plan involves the eating contract. The other is the plan devised as a result of the Psychiatric Consult. Complete the table below to include elements of the latter plan.

Psychosocial Treatment Plan	Specific interventions
Individual therapy	
Family conference/family therapy	
Relationship to eating contract	
Medication	

→ • Still in the chart, click on **Patient Education**.
  • Read the report.

7. Identify the treatment outcomes for Tiffany Sheldon. Can you think of other important outcomes?

LESSON **13** _____

Psychiatric Nursing Care of the Adolescent Patient

👓 **Reading Assignment:** Adolescent Psychiatric Nursing (Chapter 36)

Patient: Tiffany Sheldon, Pediatrics Floor, Room 305

Goal: To gain greater understanding of adolescence in order to provide psychiatric nursing care to an adolescent patient.

Objectives:

• Understand the developmental stage of adolescence.
• Explore select theoretical views of adolescence.
• Identify key areas to be included when assessing the adolescent patient.
• Explore maladaptive responses seen in adolescence.
• Describe nursing interventions effective in working with adolescents.
• Explore the nurse's own issues when working with adolescent patients.
• Evaluate treatment outcomes for an adolescent patient.

Exercise 1

 Clinical Preparation: Writing Activity

🕐 30 minutes

1. Adolescence is a time of transition characterized by _____ and

_____. During this period, there is also a shift in _____ and

_____.

2. During adolescence there are several important tasks to be accomplished before transitioning into adulthood. List these tasks below.

3. Developmental tasks of adolescence are described in a variety of theories, from biological to multidimensional. Using the multidimensional theory, discuss adolescent development.

4. When doing an assessment, the nurse must include key components specific to the adolescent patient, always checking for high-risk problems. Place an X next to components that would be important to include for this special population.

   _____ a. Appearance

   _____ b. Growth and development

   _____ c. Parent and family health

   _____ d. Emotional and physical status

   _____ e. Coping and interaction patterns

   _____ f. Activities of daily living

   _____ g. Perception of health

   _____ h. Family life

5. Adolescents think and worry about many issues. Issues typical of most adolescents are:
   a. body image.
   b. identity.
   c. independence.
   d. social role.
   e. sexual behavior.
   f. all of the above.

6. Body image, identity, and independence are three of the issues that can produce adaptive or maladaptive responses as the adolescent attempts to cope with the developmental tasks at hand. Match these issues and characteristics.

Adolescent Issue	**Characteristics**
_____ Body image	a. Seen as being free of parental control; seeks out adult situations; can become frightened and overwhelmed in the process
_____ Identity	
_____ Independence	b. Growth and development varies widely; growth is uneven and sudden; compares self to peers
	c. Childhood dreams end; becomes negative and contrary; can feel isolated, lonely, and confused

7. There are three types of parenting styles that can help/hinder independence and autonomy in the adolescent. Complete the table below by describing the characteristics of each style and indicating whether the style helps or hinders adolescent autonomy.

Parenting Style	Characteristics	Help or Hinder?
Traditional		
Authoritarian		
Democratic		

8. Maladaptive responses in adolescence include a variety of behaviors. Discuss the maladaptive responses of depression and body image.

Exercise 2

 CD-ROM Activity

 30 minutes

- Sign in to work at Pacific View Regional Hospital on the Obstetrics Floor for Period of Care 3. (*Note:* If you are already in the virtual hospital from a previous exercise, click on **Leave the Floor** and then **Restart the Program** to get to the sign-in window.)
- Select Tiffany Sheldon in Room 305.
- Click on **Go to Nurses' Station**.
- Click on **Chart** and then on **305.**
- Click on and review the following chart sections: **History and Physical**, **Nursing Admission**, **Mental Health**, and **Consultations**.

1. In working with adolescents, the nurse must be able to distinguish between age-expected behavior and maladaptive responses. Based on your review of Tiffany Sheldon's chart, complete the table below.

Issues in Adolescence	Age-Expected Behavior	Maladaptive Response
Body image		
Mood		
Activity		

2. The specific problems of adolescence that make Tiffany Sheldon a high-risk adolescent are:
   a. substance use and truancy.
   b. severe eating disorder and depressed mood.
   c. suicidal and self-injurious behavior.
   d. problems with conduct and violence.
   e. anxiety and sexual promiscuity.

3. The nurse must understand a few basic principles when working with adolescents. Place an X next to the actions that represent the nurse's understanding of these principles in working with Tiffany Sheldon.

   _____ a. Meet individually with patient to form an alliance and gain her perspective

   _____ b. Provide health information about healthy and unhealthy adolescent activities

   _____ c. Provide adolescent with only written health information since she will be too embarrassed to listen to verbal information

   _____ d. Educate adolescent on normal teen behaviors

   _____ e. Only meet with the adolescent together with the parents

   _____ f. Help adolescent to build healthy coping skills to deal with stress

4. Considering the psychological aspects of Tiffany Sheldon's maladaptive responses, discuss the type of therapy suggested in the Psychiatric Consult and the rationale for each therapy.

5. Can you think of any of your own unresolved issues regarding adolescence that might arise in working with a patient such as Tiffany Sheldon? Explain.

6. The nurse must evaluate objectively the nursing care that has been provided to Tiffany Sheldon and her family. List the important questions to ask in determining whether she and her family have met the treatment goals outlined in the treatment plan.

Evaluation of Psychiatric Nursing Care

LESSON 14

Geropsychiatric Nursing

 Reading Assignment: Geropsychiatric Nursing (Chapter 37)

Patient: Kathryn Doyle, Skilled Nursing Floor, Room 503

Goal: To understand, assess, and care for geriatric patients.

Objectives:

- Identify symptoms of mental illness in the elderly.
- Discuss theories of aging from a variety of perspectives.
- Understand necessary skills of the geropsychiatric nurse.
- Acknowledge biases in working with the elderly patient.
- Provide a comprehensive assessment of the geriatric patient.
- Identify common responses elderly people have in relation to the aging process.
- Plan and coordinate the care for a geriatric patient.
- Know effective treatment strategies to use with the geriatric patient and their family.
- Evaluate the care given to the geriatric patient.

Exercise 1

 Clinical Preparation: Writing Activity

15 minutes

1. Mental illness in the elderly may be underestimated and left undiagnosed because the symptoms may be attributed to _____, _____, _____, or the lack of _____ diagnostic criteria. For example, mental illnesses such as _____ are often misdiagnosed or undertreated.

2. Mental health in late life depends on a number of factors. Select the factors that apply.
   a. Physiological and psychological status
   b. Economic resources
   c. Social support systems
   d. Personality
   e. Typical lifestyle
   f. All of the above

3. The biological, psychological, and sociocultural theories of aging provide ways of defining aging and help to explain the causes and consequences of the aging process. Complete the table below by summarizing the three theories.

Theory of Aging	Summary of Theory
Biological	
Psychological	
Sociocultural	

4. Describe the necessary skills of the geropsychiatric nurse.

5. _____ is an especially effective approach to providing for the biopsychosocial needs of the elderly.

6. Discuss possible biases you may have in working with the geriatric population.

Exercise 2

 CD-ROM Activity

 45 minutes

- Sign in to work at Pacific View Regional Hospital on the Skilled Nursing Floor for Period of Care 2. (*Note:* If you are already in the virtual hospital from a previous exercise, click on **Leave the Floor** and then **Restart the Program** to get to the sign-in window.)
- Select Kathryn Doyle in Room 503.
- Click on **Go to Nurses' Station**.
- Click on **Chart** and then on **503**.
- Click on and read the **History and Physical**.
- Click on **Consultations** and read the Psychiatric Clinical Nurse Specialist Consult.

1. Kathryn Doyle has one of the four Ds of geropsychiatric assessment. Identify which one she has and discuss the need to include this "D" in a geropsychiatric assessment.

2. Kathryn Doyle seems to be experiencing anxiety. Which of these statements are true regarding anxiety in the elderly?

_____ a. Comorbid anxiety and depression are common in the elderly.

_____ b. All types of anxiety combined are more prevalent than depression in the elderly.

_____ c. Untreated anxiety can contribute to sleep problems, cognitive impairments, and decreased quality of life.

_____ d. Anxiety does not affect the family.

_____ e. Antianxiety medications also decrease depression.

3. Besides interviewing the geriatric patient and completing a mental status, there are other key components of the geropsychiatric nursing assessment. Complete the table below to include data specific to Kathryn Doyle.

Component	Key Elements	Assessment of Kathryn Doyle
Behavioral responses		
Functional abilities		
Physiological responses		
Social support		

- Click on **Return to 503**.
- Click on **Patient Care**.
- Click on **Nurse-Client Interactions**.
- Select and view the video titled **1150: Depression—Cause, Treatment**. (*Note:* If this video is not available, check the virtual clock to see whether enough time has elapsed. The video cannot be viewed before its specified time.)

4. Depression and sadness are sometimes viewed as a normal part of aging. Kathryn Doyle's response to life events that have occurred over the past 9 months has resulted in a disturbance in her mood. Place an X next to each correct statement as it pertains to normal sadness, grief, and loss in the elderly.

_____ a. Depression, grief, and loss are common in later life.

_____ b. Prolonged grief and mourning needs to be treated.

_____ c. Death of a life partner can compound the cumulative loses of aging.

_____ d. The loss of hope by elders with disabilities may result from or cause a depressive reaction.

_____ e. Common symptoms of depression include decreased appetite and weight loss.

_____ f. Fatigue, apathy, and loss of interest in friends and usual activities are symptoms of depression.

→ • Click on **MAR**.
 • Review Kathryn Doyle's medication list.

5. Does Kathryn Doyle have medication ordered to treat her depression? Discuss the role of medication to treat depression in the elderly.

6. Based on the nurse's assessment, Kathryn Doyle has other affective, somatic, stress, and behavioral responses common to the elderly. Complete the table below by outlining her specific issues associated with these common reactions.

Response	Type of Response	Issues Involved with Kathryn Doyle's Response
Affective	Situational low self-esteem	
Somatic	Imbalanced nutrition	
Stress	Relocation stress syndrome	
Behavioral	Social isolation	

→ • Click on **Return to Nurses' Station**.

 • Click on **Leave the Floor**.

 • Click on **Restart the Program**.

 • Sign in to work at Pacific View Regional Hospital on the Skilled Nursing Floor for Period of Care 3. Again, select Kathryn Doyle as your patient.

 • Click on **Go to Nurses' Station**.

 • Click on Room **503** at the bottom of the screen.

 • Click on **Patient Care**.

 • Click on **Nurse-Client Interactions**.

 • Select and view the video titled **1505: Assessment—Elder Abuse**. (*Note:* If this video is not available, check the virtual clock to see whether enough time has elapsed. The video cannot be viewed before its specified time.)

7. Elder neglect and abuse has become more common in our society as elderly people no longer have the status and respect they once had through their extended families. Serving as the patient's advocate, the nurse must be on alert for signs of elder neglect, abuse, or exploitation. What are the signs that Kathryn Doyle is being neglected, exploited, or abused?

8. During the family conference the issue of theft will be addressed. Another concern that needs to be discussed is Kathryn Doyle continuing to live in her son's home post hip fracture. If this living arrangement is to work, the environment must include several basic characteristics therapeutic for elderly patients. Place an X next to the critical elements that must be included in the environment.

_____ a. Sense of calm and quiet

_____ b. Structured routine (based on the elder's usual lifestyle)

_____ c. Consistent physical layout

_____ d. Activities that produce cognitive stimulation

_____ e. Safe environment

_____ f. Personal items that provide familiarity and a sense of security

_____ g. Focus on strengths and abilities

9. Most elders (about 80%) are cared for in the home. What topics should the nurse include in family education and support sessions that would be critical to Kathryn Doyle's recovery and future?

10. Aftercare for elderly patients is often necessary for a successful treatment outcome. After discharge what agency support do you think Kathryn Doyle's son will need in the care of his mother in the home?

LESSON 15 —————

Care of Survivors of Abuse and Violence

👓 **Reading Assignment:** Care of Survivors of Abuse and Violence (Chapter 38)

Patient: Dorothy Grant, Obstetrics Floor, Room 201

Goal: To care for a patient who is a survivor of abuse and violence.

Objectives:

- Identify characteristics of someone who has experienced abuse or violence.
- Define characteristics common to violent families.
- Understand the difference between myths and realities associated with survivors of abuse.
- Compare and contrast the Paternalistic Model and the Empowerment Model of intervention in relation to battered women.
- Describe strengths and coping strategies of someone who is experiencing abuse or violence.
- Discuss nursing assessment and interventions using the Empowerment Model.
- Identify central themes in abusive relationships.
- Understand common barriers to battered spouses leaving an abusive relationship.
- Describe critical elements of a discharge plan of someone who is being abused.

Exercise 1

 Clinical Preparation: Writing Activity

 15 minutes

1. In describing someone who has experienced abuse or violence, provide a rationale using the term *survivor* rather than *victim*.

2. Factors common to violent families include which of the following?
    a. Multigenerational family process
    b. Owning and keeping weapons in the home
    c. Social isolation
    d. Use and abuse of power
    e. Alcohol and drug abuse
    f. All except b

3. There are several myths regarding survivors of abuse. Complete the table below by describing the reality associated with the myths listed.

Myth	Reality
Abused spouses can end the violence by divorcing their abuser.	
The victim can learn to stop doing things that provoke the violence.	
Pregnancy protects a woman from being battered.	
Abused women tacitly accept the abuse by trying to conceal it, not reporting it, or failing to seek help.	

4. The attitudes that nurses bring to the health care setting shape their responses toward survivors of violence. Place an X next to each true statement.

_____ a. Nurses may blame the survivor if behavior leading up to the abuse was questionable.

_____ b. Nurses have difficulty understanding why a battered woman does not leave her abuser.

_____ c. Nurses always believe that people get what they deserve.

_____ d. Nurses may offer advice and sympathy instead of respect.

_____ e. The more the patient resembles the nurse, the easier it is for the nurse to recognize violence.

_____ f. More nurses have been victimized by violence than any other work group.

_____ g. Nurses need to forget about their own experiences with violence.

_____ h. Nurses who have had clinical experiences with survivors of violence may be less blaming than nurses who have not.

5. What is your attitude about domestic violence and how is it shaped?

Exercise 2

 CD-Rom Activity

15 minutes

- Sign in to work at Pacific View Regional Hospital on the Obstetrics Floor for Period of Care 2. (*Note:* If you are already in the virtual hospital from a previous exercise, click on **Leave the Floor** and then **Restart the Program** to get to the sign-in window.)
- Select Dorothy Grant, Room 201.
- Click on **Go to Nurses' Station**.
- Click on **Chart** and then on **201**.
- To answer questions 1 through 6, review the following sections of Dorothy Grant's chart: **Nursing Admission, Mental Health**, and **Consultations**. (*Hint:* In the Mental Health section, read the Psychiatric/Mental Health Assessment; then scroll down to review the Abuse Screening.)

1. Listed below are the five forms of abuse within families that reflect domestic struggles for power and control. Place an X next to the forms of abuse Dorothy Grant is experiencing.

_____ a. Physical

_____ b. Sexual

_____ c. Emotional

_____ d. Psychological

_____ e. Economic

2. Dorothy Grant is a member of one of the special populations that are vulnerable to abuse. These include children, the elderly, and developmentally disabled, as well as

_____. The most widespread form of family violence is

_____.

3. There are general characteristics of violent families; these are listed in the left column below. In the right column, identify any specific characteristics of Dorothy Grant's family that correspond to the general characteristics of violent families.

Characteristic of Violent Families	Dorothy Grant's Family Characteristics
Multigenerational transmission	
Social isolation	
Use and abuse of power	
Alcohol and drug abuse	

4. What are Dorothy Grant's strengths in dealing with her abusive situation?

5. What are her coping strategies in dealing with her abusive relationship?

6. Depression is a common response by women in abusive relationships. According to

Dorothy Grant's depression scale, her level of depression is _____.

Exercise 3

 CD-ROM Activity

30 minutes

- Sign in to work at Pacific View Regional Hospital on the Obstetrics Floor for Period of Care 2. (*Note:* If you are already in the virtual hospital from a previous exercise, click on **Leave the Floor** and then **Restart the Program** to get to the sign-in window.)
- Select Dorothy Grant, Room 201.
- Click on **Go to Nurses' Station**.
- Click on Room **201** at the bottom of the screen.
- Click on **Patient Care** and then on **Nurse-Client Interactions**.
- Select and view the video titled **1115: Nurse-Patient Communication**. (*Note:* If this video is not available, check the virtual clock to see whether enough time has elapsed. The video cannot be viewed before its specified time.)

1. The Empowerment Model of intervention has been found to be very effective in working with battered women. The basic principles of this model are listed below. In the video clip you just viewed, the nurse used the Empowerment Model when interacting with Dorothy Grant. In the right column below, cite specific examples of statements made by the nurse that correspond to the Empowerment Model's principles. (*Note:* You may add suggestions of what the nurse could have said to support the Empowerment Model if you think there is room for improvement.)

Empowerment Model	Nurse's Statements
There is a mutual sharing of knowledge and information.	
The nurse strategizes with the survivor.	
Survivors are helped to recognize societal influences.	
The survivor's competence and experience are respected.	

2. The nurse uses other therapeutic responses when interacting with Dorothy Grant. These are listed in the right column below. Match each response to the technique it utilizes.

Technique	**Nurse's Response**
_____ Mutual goal-sharing	a. Shows active listening responses such as "Feeling scared is a perfectly normal reaction."
_____ Focusing	
_____ Using broad open-ended questions	b. "The clinical nurse specialist and the social worker work together to identify your immediate needs."
_____ Listening	
	c. "Right now your first priority is you own well-being and the well-being of your children."
	d. "Would you like to talk about your concerns now?"; "Is there anything I can do to help?"

3. The immediate goal of the nurse in working with Dorothy Grant is to develop trust. In order to develop trust, the nurse must express nonjudgmental listening and psychological support. How did the nurse accomplish or not accomplish this in the video?

4. What are the constraints that will make it difficult for Dorothy Grant to leave her husband?
   a. Still in love with her husband
   b. Lack of housing and financial resources
   c. Her church's support of marriage
   d. Societal stigma
   e. Domestic violence reporting not mandatory in any state
   f. Husband in jail
   g. b and c

5. Dorothy Grant has left her husband twice before and returned. For the battered woman, what are the three main purposes of this behavior?

6. One of the most frightening realities Dorothy Grant may face in leaving her husband is

   _____.

7. Several themes expressed by women in abusive relationships have been identified. Knowing the themes Dorothy Grant is expressing will help the nurse in assessing and planning interventions. Identify Dorothy Grant's themes below.

Themes of Women Who Have Been in Abusive Relationships	Dorothy Grant's Themes
Lack of relational authenticity	
Immobility	
Emptiness	
Disconnection	

8. Discharge planning will be crucial for Dorothy Grant. Place an X next to any activities that will be necessary for a successful outcome.

   _____ a. Create a Safety Planning Checklist

   _____ b. Provide her with survivors of abuse and violence hotline phone numbers

   _____ c. Find supportive alternate living arrangement for Dorothy Grant and her children

9. Discuss your own thoughts about Dorothy Grant's current and past responses to the abuse. Do you think she has responded in the way a typical person would react to incredible physical and emotional trauma? Or do you believe her responses have been more pathological in nature? Explain.

Notes:

Notes:

Notes:

Notes:

Notes:

Notes:

Notes: